CW01149565

BEING WELL

HOW TO ACTIVATE YOUR SEVEN HEALING SUPERPOWERS

SONIA MARIE ROMERO

Copyright © 2024 Sonia Marie Romero.

Cover Design by Olga Jane Tanud-tanud
Cover Photo by Laura Burbano @thecreative18

All rights reserved. No part of this book may be reproduced, stored, or transmitted by any means—whether auditory, graphic, mechanical, or electronic—without written permission of both publisher and author, except in the case of brief excerpts used in critical articles and reviews. Unauthorized reproduction of any part of this work is illegal and is punishable by law.

ISBN: 979-8-89419-515-5 (sc)
ISBN: 979-8-89419-516-2 (hc)
ISBN: 979-8-89419-517-9 (e)

Because of the dynamic nature of the Internet, any web addresses or links contained in this book may have changed since publication and may no longer be valid. The views expressed in this work are solely those of the author and do not necessarily reflect the views of the publisher, and the publisher hereby disclaims any responsibility for them.

THE EWINGS PUBLISHING

One Galleria Blvd., Suite 1900, Metairie, LA 70001
(504) 702-6708

CONTENTS

Acknowledgements v
Foreword vii
Introduction ix

Part One: Your Seven Healing Superpowers 1

Chapter 1 I'm Not Crazy 3
Chapter 2 Three Hats Are Enough 11
Chapter 3 Four Chins 21
Chapter 4 Beauty Really is an Inside Job 31
Chapter 5 You Are Much More Than What You Eat 41
Chapter 6 Move It Or Lose It 53
Chapter 7 How to Manage Our Cravings 63

Part Two: Becoming Healthy 79

Chapter 8   Trust Your Intuition 81
Chapter 9   The Self Care Mindset 89
Chapter 10 Your Body's Natural Detoxification System 101
Chapter 11 Healing Our Gut 111
Chapter 12 Balancing Our Hormones 121
Chapter 13 Commitment To Health 131
Chapter 14 Relationships That Nurture Our Wellbeing 139

Part Three: Becoming Well 151

Chapter 15 Savory Recipes 153
Chapter 16 Sweet Can Be Good 161
Chapter 17 Recipes For Life 167

ACKNOWLEDGEMENTS

As I stand on the threshold of presenting this book to the world, my heart swells with gratitude and profound appreciation. This writing journey has been nothing short of extraordinary, and I am humbled beyond words by the incredible support, unwavering love, and boundless encouragement that have helped me to bring this vision to life.

To my cherished clients: you are the heartbeat of this book. Your trust in me, your commitment to your well-being, and your unyielding dedication to embracing holistic nutrition as a path to optimal health have been a constant source of inspiration. Each step you've taken on your healing journey has fueled my own passion to share the transformative power of holistic practices with the world. Your stories, triumphs, and perseverance are woven into the fabric of these pages, and I am profoundly grateful for the privilege of walking alongside you.

My family are my rock and my foundation. Laffit, Jacob, Joshua, and Tori, you have been my unwavering pillars of strength. From the late-night writing sessions to the moments of doubt, you've been my guiding light, offering boundless love and support. Your belief in me, your encouragement, and your willingness to lend a hand in whatever capacity needed, have been the wind beneath my hummingbird wings. This book is a testament to the values you've instilled in me and the deep connections we share.

To my mentors, fellow practitioners, and countless friends: your wisdom, support, and expertise have been invaluable. Tamilee, Gina, Melanie, Maria, Bobbie, Elyssa, the list goes on and on. Your willingness to share insights, answer questions, and offer guidance have been instrumental in shaping the content of this book. Your collective dedication to holistic well-being has created a community that constantly uplifts and inspires me.

I extend my gratitude to my family members who have been part of this journey in ways both seen and unseen. Jacqui, Wendy, Kevin, Lisa, Debbi, Blake, Albert, David, Mom, and those that are no longer with us Dad & Tammy. To all my beautiful nieces and nephews. Trevor, Tristan, Krista, Rebecca, Madison, Morgan, Hunter and Andyn.

A special note of appreciation goes to Will T Wilkinson, my writing coach and editor, who polished these words and played a crucial role in bringing this vision to fruition. His unwavering belief in the power of holistic well-being sparked the initial idea for this book. Will, your keen insights and attention to detail have enriched the content and elevated its credibility. Your enthusiasm, encouragement, and unflagging support have been a driving force throughout this process; I could not have completed a lifelong dream of writing this book without you.

Lastly, I offer my heartfelt gratitude to each reader who embarks on this holistic journey of being well with an open heart and a curious mind. May this book serve as a guiding light on your path to wellness, and may its pages resonate with the same love, support, and empowerment that have fueled its creation.

In closing, this book stands as a collective endeavor, a tapestry woven with threads of connection, dedication, and a shared commitment to well-being. From the depths of my heart, I thank everyone who has played a role in making this dream a reality. May the wisdom within these pages empower you to embrace a new way towards health and to activate your seven healing superpowers, in a profound and transformative journey towards a life of radiant health and well-being.

With boundless gratitude,

Sonia Marie Romero

FOREWORD

BEING WELL is not just another book; it's a beacon of hope, knowledge, and inspiration.

You're about to take an incredible journey with Sonia Marie Romero, a remarkable woman and my dear friend. In this, her debut book, Sonia shares her transformative story that will touch your heart and ignite your passion for self-improvement. And I know this reading adventure will inspire and empower you to activate your own seven healing superpowers.

As a close friend of Sonia's for nearly three decades, I found myself captivated by her words in this profound book, even though I thought I knew her story inside out. BEING WELL drew me in and awakened emotions that compelled me to reflect on my own journey of activating my healing superpowers.

I loved all the inspiring quotes in BEING WELL that ignite the mind, nourish the soul, and offer inspiring perspectives on wellness. My favorite is the one from David Wolfe: *"True beauty comes from the inside out; it emerges from proper thinking as well as proper nutrition and exercise."* So true and what a great reminder!

As a renowned fitness professional who has helped thousands of individuals achieve better health and wellness, I already possess extensive knowledge in this field. But there are times when all of us are just too close to our struggles to find the solutions.

This is where having a coach becomes invaluable, someone who holds us accountable and guides us toward the answers we seek. Reading

BEING WELL has reminded me of the importance of seeking support, especially when we believe that we know it all!

My own greatest health challenge has been my gut and it's an area where I've definitely struggled to find a resolution. Sonia's insights have shed light on new perspectives, with practical advice and strategies to address my gut health concerns.

Join Sonia on this transformative journey to discover the power within to activate your seven healing superpowers. Become what Sonia calls a "client by book" and let her voice guide you toward a healed, vital, resilient, and well-being-filled life.

This book will be a gift to all my clients. I will encourage them to use it to unlock their true potential for creating a healthy, happy life and to help their families and friends do the same.

Tamilee Webb

Fitness Star of Buns of Steel

INTRODUCTION

"Health is a state of complete mental, social and physical well-being, not merely the absence of disease or infirmity."

—World Health Organization, 1948

Welcome! How I wish we were meeting in person, sitting in my office here in Southern California, sharing my favorite subject - holistic health. I'd listen carefully to learn about your concerns. I'd ask questions about your health history, your lifestyle, current challenges, and your healing priorities.

Then I would introduce you to something you probably wouldn't have ever heard about before, which is also the theme of this book: your seven healing superpowers. We all have them, but no-one has educated us to know it or to know how to use them. That's what you would learn if you became my client. It's what you will learn as you read this book.

When we think of superpowers we probably think of superheroes. And... that's not us! We can't fly or bend steel or see through walls. That's OK. These superpowers are different. For starters, everyone has them. And that doesn't mean that we're all mutants! These superpowers are normal, we're born with them. But we rarely learn how to activate them.

A second difference is that we don't use them competitively. While superheroes wield their powers to defeat bad guys, we use ours to heal ourselves. The final difference – which is the most important one to understand, is that we're already using them... we just don't realize it. So, think about what happens when you cut your finger. It starts to heal, immediately. You keep the wound clean, maybe put a bandage on it, or get stitches if it's serious. But we understand that there's a healing power in our bodies doing the actual repair work. No doctor does that. Drugs, surgery, therapy… whatever we might use just supports that healing power to work its magic. And it *is* magic! It's keeping our hearts beating 24/7. Incredible!

> *You can activate these seven superpowers*
> *to heal yourself and life will never be the same.*

Who Are You?

We've all heard the phrase: "You are what you eat." If that's true, it may explain why so many of us are stressed out and unhappy. But I tell my clients:

> *"You are what you eat … and you are also what you eat eats."*
> *Now, that's sobering. What's fed to our food? It's in there, we're eating it!*

"The United States has a bad reputation when it comes to healthy diets. That's because at least a third of Americans enjoy fast food on any given day. The United States is the biggest fast-food consumer on the globe. One-third of children 2 to 19 years old and two-thirds of U.S. adults are obese or overweight. Recent data suggests that just 10% of American adults meet the veggie requirements."[1]

I see the results of this every day. I've been coaching in the health and wellness world for 31 years. Clients often show up for help in losing weight or dealing with one or two symptoms. I introduce them to the wide world of holistic health which is about so much more than looking

---

[1] https://www.bensnaturalhealth.com/blog/general-health/average-american-diet-and-exercise/#:~:text=2%2C000%20for%20women.-,Does%20the%20Average%20American%20Have%20a%20Healthy%20Diet%3F,and%2022%25%20from%20added%20sugars.

good and treating symptoms. And I help them discover and harness their healing superpowers.

> *"By choosing healthy over skinny you are choosing self-love over self-judgement."*
>
> —Steve Maraboli.

I am certified and experienced in these areas of health:

- Owner and chef of "The Cajun Way Café"
- Holistic Health Coach and Wellness Counselor, IIN
- Functional Medicine Chef
- Psychology of Eating
- Food Matters Health Coach
- GT5P -Gut Healing practitioner
- Miss Fitness USA competitor
- AFAA Certified personal trainer
- ACE Certified Life Coach and Aerobics Instructor
- I've studied over 100 dietary theories.

I'm writing this book because I've had first-hand, dramatic, personal experience of healing from serious diseases (yes, more than one) and I'm passionate about healing our bodies with these seven healing superpowers. I love helping my clients reverse disease and take control over their health and daily habits. But I can only see so many people in my personal practice. By writing out my experience in this book, I'm making myself available to thousands of people who need health coaching, people who would never be able to find me and learn from me.

I'll be sharing with you what I share with my clients, how to activate these seven healing superpowers to improve your physical, mental, emotional, and spiritual wellbeing.

Who are you? The one who will be doing that!

Getting Set

As we begin our healing journey together, I invite you to pause for a moment to establish your mindset. We don't usually think about this, but attitude affects everything. In fact, attitude even affects our digestion. Did you know that? If we eat when we're angry we might get bloated, suffer acid reflux, even develop diarrhea. Our attitude also affects the quality of the food we are preparing for our family.

Many indigenous tribes considered food preparation a ritual event. The Lakota people still teach their children about this. "During these special meetings, elder women and "master teachers" gather with young women to learn and share the protocol, ceremony, and logistical techniques of making these foods. For many of the women and girls present, these gatherings are their first introduction to the art of preparing these most sacred foods."[2]

My writing coach told me about attending a tea ceremony in Kyoto, Japan and how the tea was served in ritual silence and how deeply emotional this felt, to honor what was being put into the body with such reverence. We've lost touch with these traditions in the era of fast-food convenience, but we can bring them back in a modern way.

In an ETimes blog, Lifestyle coach Luke Coutinho talks about what happens in our bodies when we are angry and stressed out while we eat. "You don't have the right kind of bacteria to break down the food you eat and even swallowing becomes difficult due to contraction of muscles. Our body will not be able to digest the food and absorb the nutrients," he added."Another reason to avoid it is because you are more prone to overeating. Our gut and brain communicate with each other all the time. But when we are angry, the communication is blocked. So, the brain does not get the signal from the gut when the stomach is full.

"The third and most important reason is that our intestine barrier, which prevents the gut bacteria from entering the bloodstream gets

---

[2] https://www.sacredhealingcircle.org/copy-of-ancient-horse-of-the-americ

weak. "Due to this, the bacteria enter the bloodstream and leads to various health complications," he explained."[3]

Why the Attitude?

I've chosen to introduce my book this way because over the decades of working with clients, I've become convinced that attitude IS the most important factor that influences our health. But that word covers a lot of territory. Consider this following short list and notice your attitude as you read, especially if you encounter something you don't immediately agree with.

- Preparing food is significant, not menial.
- Our attitude in the kitchen affects the quality and flavor of the food.
- Who we are shows up in the food we create.
- Our dishes can become works of art, even if it's just a sandwich.
- Our attitude influences the choices we make, which determines our behaviors and how we continue to develop ourselves (or not).
- Ongoing personal development requires being honest and doing deep "work."
- Power ultimately comes from the way you think…ie your attitude.

Some authors preach to their readers who become passive spectators, just taking in the information. That's not me. I get engaged with my clients and I want to engage with you. This means that I'll be inviting you to participate with me throughout this book, with worksheets, recipes, stories… Most of all, I invite you to explore the seven superpowers I've

---

[3] https://timesofindia.indiatimes.com/life-style/health-fitness/health-news/why-you-should-never-eat-food-when-you-are-angry-or-anxious/articleshow/77759723.cms

identified, learn how to access and activate them, and enjoy experimenting in the kitchen and in your life.

Mindset, what we've just been exploring, is the number one priority.

Your Seven Healing Superpowers

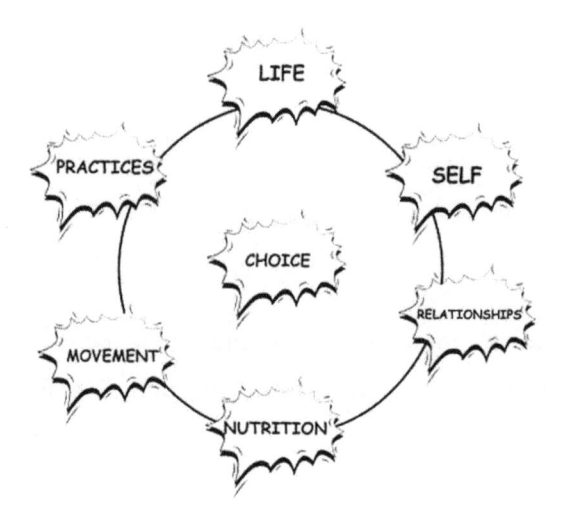

(Diagram: a circle of seven bursts labeled LIFE, SELF, RELATIONSHIPS, NUTRITION, MOVEMENT, PRACTICES, with CHOICE in the center.)

People may disagree on many things, including what food to eat and how to stay healthy, but there's one thing that's beyond argument: we're alive. We're alive and something is keeping our hearts beating. There's no wire, no battery, and we're not consciously doing it ourselves. This introduces our first superpower, life itself. Life is in control of our bodies, right? If we cut our finger, it heals on its own. We're wise to keep the wound clean, maybe put on a bandage, but the life force in our body does the healing.

Our attitude either supports or suppresses this superpower.

Our second superpower is ourselves. You. Me. Every individual is unique and has different needs for being healthy and happy.

But I'm referring to our relationship with ourselves. Self-esteem issues can be a big problem. They can make us sick. The voice in our head and our negative self-talk is vital to our health.

The second superpower to access is our attitude about ourselves.

Number three is our relationship with others. Family, friendship, community… every relationship we have is either nurturing or depleting. And this affects our health. You'll be learning about relationship nutrition in a later chapter.

We are always in relationship, with others,
with circumstances, and with ourselves.

Superpower four is Choice. I put it right in the middle between the three internal powers and the three external ones that follow. All of us get to choose what we eat, what we do, how we behave. It's our choices that determine whether we are healthy or sick and also if we access and develop all these superpowers, or not.

This one the super superpower!

Superpower five is nutrition. The food we eat, is important but, is not number one. That's because of what I already mentioned about attitude. Even the best food won't give us any nutrition if we can't digest it because we're stressed out. That said, what we eat is VERY important and we'll get into the details to simplify what can be a very confusing topic.

Everything we eat is a choice and we can make healthy choices.

Superpower six is movement. I say movement rather than exercise because it's important to understand how important motion is. If we aren't moving throughout the day, our whole system gets stagnant.

So, a big yes to regular exercise but an even bigger yes to movement. If you sit a lot, as I do working with clients, it's vital to get up regularly and move. Set a timer if you need to.

As the saying goes, "move it or lose it."

The final superpower is health practices. This includes everything we can do throughout the day to stay fit, like stretching, meditating, walking in nature, etc. You'll learn about a broad range of health practices in the pages ahead.

It's what we do regularly that makes the difference.

Here they are in a convenient list:

1. Life
2. Self
3. Relationships
4. Choice
5. Nutrition
6. Movement
7. Practices

The most important thing I want to communicate is that you have the ability to help yourself to become and stay healthy. Yes, we all have challenges, including our DNA and habit patterns established in childhood. But it's never too late to make positive changes. That's what I help my clients do every day and what I'll be helping you do through these pages.

What you read can change your life forever and in the best ways imaginable. That's my hope for you and it's why I'm writing this book.

Bon voyage!

PART ONE

YOUR SEVEN HEALING SUPERPOWERS

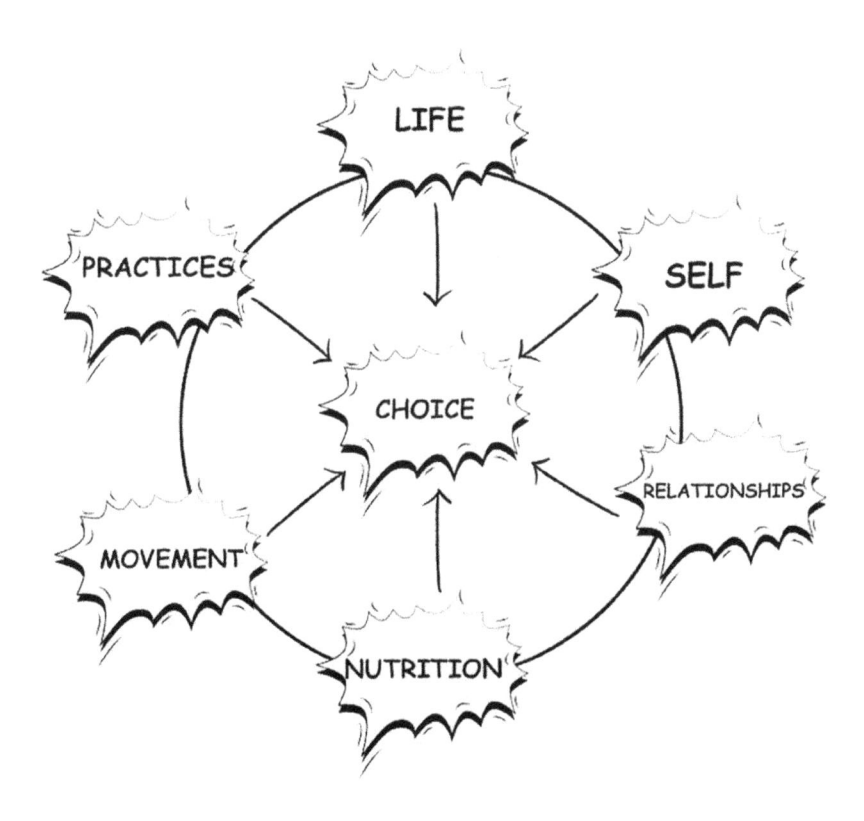

LIFE

PRACTICES

SELF

CHOICE

MOVEMENT

RELATIONSHIPS

NUTRITION

PART ONE

YOUR SEVEN HEALING SUPERPOWERS

CHAPTER 1

I'M NOT CRAZY

"One thing that makes people crazy is being told that the experiences they have did not actually happen. That the circumstances that hem them in are imaginary. That the problems are all in their head, and that if they are distressed, it is a sign of their failure. When success would be to shut up or to cease to know what they know. Out of this unbearable predicament come the rebels who choose failure and risk and the prisoners who choose compliance."

—Rebecca Solnit

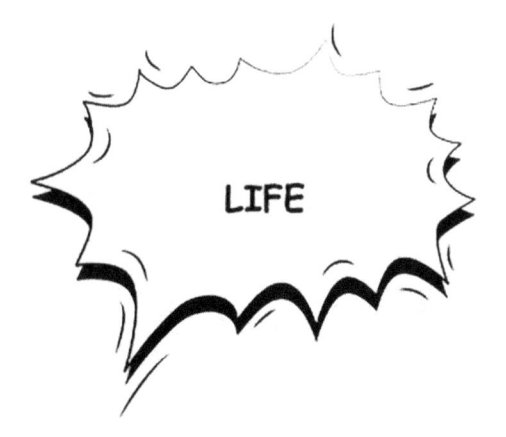

A regular client recently referred me to a friend who'd had a bone marrow transplant and was in absolute hell. She was stuck in bed, couldn't eat, broke out in a rash all over her body, had so much irritation in her mouth that she couldn't eat, had a hard time talking and couldn't sleep.

Her doctor offered her no hope and she was withering away. "There's nothing you can do," he told her. "I'm sorry. Unfortunately, you're going to die." I gave her five things she could do to improve her health. "What?" she said. "You mean, I can do something to feel better?"

That was weeks ago. She came in again the other day, with make up on, her hair done, and wearing a beautiful blouse. I said, "You look beautiful, where are you going?" She said, "I got dressed for you!"

Then she told me: "Those five things you told me to do this week? I did them all. And yesterday I got in the car for the first time in six months to go grocery shopping. My whole family are wondering, "What happened?"

She told them and she told me: "Now I have hope!"

She also told me that her rash was disappearing. She said, "You have no idea… The pain I've been in for the last two years, it's almost gone!" She mentioned that when a friend asked how her pain level was that she began to feel it again. Bingo! There's that second superpower, the way we think about what's happening to us. Attitude! Mindset! It's so important. Talking about how sick we are with someone who sympathizes with us doesn't help. (SP#2)

Now she's recovering. And she knows that it's what she's doing for herself that is making the difference. This is what I call an "everyday miracle." The same is available to everyone. There *is* hope.

What Are We Learning From Our Challenges?

"That which does not kill us makes us stronger." That's what the German philosopher Friedrich Nietzsche said two hundred years and ago and many of us have believed it. But recent studies have proven him wrong, at least some of the time.

"A study from Brown University is calling into question the validity of that statement. The researchers reported that past traumatic events usually make people more sensitive and vulnerable to future problems, not more resilient."[4]

Like you, I've experienced a considerable amount of trauma in my life. I've learned that it only makes me stronger when I learn from the experience. If I process the trauma, do my inner work as some people say, then the challenge I overcome can indeed improve my coping skills in the future. But some life traumas are so extreme that they literally reprogram us, so that it requires professional intervention to heal the wound and gain value from the ordeal.

I know something is wrong.

In fact, everything feels wrong. I'd given birth for the first time six years before and that had been scary enough, but this time is different. I stare up at the doctor and nurses and I know: I'm not just fighting for my life this time, it's my baby who is at risk.

"Sorry," I hear through a fog, "you won't be having a natural birth this time either. We have to do an emergency C-section immediately. We must take this baby out right now!"

The doctor has his hand inside me. "Come on baby, come on, come on baby," he urges. The doctor shouts at the anesthesiologist. "I need to cut her open now!"

"You can't," I hear, "she's not ready yet." I'm crying as I beg the anesthesiologist: "Please don't let him cut me open before I'm numb." Forty very long minutes go by in a blur and my precious baby is born into this world.

But something is still wrong. My baby has no heartbeat. They revive my child, it's a miracle, and the nurse announces, "Congratulations, you have a girl!" I instantly feel sick. No. No! I murmur to my husband, "I felt like it was going to be a boy," I say. Now I feel like a horrible mother, rejecting

---

[4] https://www.linkedin.com/pulse/why-expression-what-doesnt-kill-you-makes-stronger-may-ray-williams?trk=pulse-article_more-articles_related-content-card

my baby this way. I should be happy, now we have a boy and a girl, this should be perfect. Moments go by and I accept it: we have a girl. Her name will be Brianna Marie, I'll give her my middle name.

But I don't feel connected to this baby, even though she is my second miracle. "You're lucky to be alive after your first delivery," the doctor tells me. "Now you have two kids. But this is your last pregnancy, Sonia."

They whisk Brianna away for tests and several hours later the pediatrician walks in. Her voice sounds odd. "I need to tell you something," she begins, "but I think your husband should be here."

She didn't make it! That's my first thought. I start sobbing but the nurse says "No, no, your baby is ok." Now I'm confused. "What," I ask, "tell me now, what is it? I can't wait for my husband to get here."

The doctor glances away nervously for a moment, then turns, her eyes wide. "I'm not sure how to tell you this. Your baby's testicles just dropped."

I gave birth to a beautiful baby boy. My intuition had been right. But the LA Times had already announced that we had a girl. And 35,000 people at Santa Anita racetrack had heard this. It became a circus, A photographer posed as a florist to deliver flowers to my room and take a photo of the baby. (SP#1) My then husband was quite famous.

Six months later, the real lessons began. I had noticed something about my Jacob. I told his pediatrician that he wasn't reacting properly to his environment. Sounds, smells ... he just was very sensitive to some things and not at all to others.

No one listened to me. No one. Two doctors, four specialists, and countless frustrating conversations later, my in-laws visited, and I heard them tell my husband, "I think she needs to go see someone... why does she think there's something wrong with the baby... Is she going crazy?"

No one is listening to me.

Yes, I was constantly telling the doctors, my family, friends, and anyone who would listen that something was wrong with Jacob. "I don't think he can hear," I told them, "And he's always throwing himself upside down."

Every doctor said the same thing: "Stop comparing him to your first born, they are completely different, there's nothing wrong with him. Maybe you should rest. Here's a number if you want to call this therapist."

They just kept doing the same ridiculous test. They showed Jacob a tool and then made it vibrate bring it near his ear. He would look at it, proving to them that he was hearing just fine. But what baby is *not* going to look at whatever is being held next to his ear?

Jacob was 13 months old when I finally got through to one of our doctors. I had him sit in a chair facing Jacob. I walked behind him where Jacob couldn't see and yelled so loud that the doctor almost fell off his stool. Jacob didn't move. It worked. The doctor agreed, maybe we needed to do some hearing tests.

Finally. We discovered that Jacob is profoundly deaf.

Trust Your Gut

A mother knows best. We do. We have intuition. "This is my baby, he came out of my body, we have a special bond. I feel what the experts Can't."

Sure, they are smarter than we are and what they know is based in science. So, it's easy for those educated voices to speak louder than ours, for us to give up searching for answers to questions they won't hear, because people will begin to think we're crazy.

We're not crazy. I'm not crazy.

There's a bigger voice within us and it speaks from love. It's a sense of knowing that can never fit inside some kind of a constructed box. The feeling doesn't stop because we get tired of hearing that everything is ok, it stops when we are heard, respected, when we feel peace in our souls because we have our answer and can move forward now. " Some people listen and some people hear".

When you feel that ease and joy and peace, move towards that feeling. Conversely, when you feel resistance towards rushing into a decision, know that this is not right for you, that you need to pause and find something else. Mothers know safety, we know what we like and don't like and we know if we want to do something or not. Once we start compromising on what we know, drifting away from what our souls want, we are also losing touch with our true self.

This introduces Superpower Number One: Life. That's what's speaking to us in those moments of clarity. And it's the most powerful force in the universe. Obviously, because it's beating our hearts and steering the stars and everything else… all at the same time. But that's all unconscious. Accessing and deploying this superpower is about becoming conscious of what's been unconscious, deliberately paying attention to what Life is trying to tell us.

> *The more we listen, the more we invest in this conscious relationship, the more of an ally Life will be.*

I once had a client; we'll call her Sally. Sally came to me suffering from breast cancer and we started off with my standard health history consultation. We discussed her general health, current medications, and her symptoms from chemo and radiation.

My intuition kicked in and I asked her how would she feel about working with me to heal her body without considering a different diet. We're just going to talk, I said. She looked at me like I was crazy (but I'm not!).

"Don't you practice holistic nutrition for healing?" she asked.

I said, "Yes, but I don't think that's what you need right now. I think you have a story that needs to be heard."

Sally must have trusted her own intuition because she agreed. This began twice monthly meetings in my office for 90-minute conversations.

The first day she arrived with one arm in a sling, on the side where her breast had been removed. She couldn't move the arm and it had been this way for three weeks. She told me how the doctors and her family all thought she should be in bed and not moving that arm.

I asked her, "Do you want to move your arm?" She said yes. I said, "What else do you want?" The healing began. Each time she voiced what she wanted; I would test her mobility by asking her to lift her arm. Before she left that first session, she could lift her arm even with her shoulder.

At one point, using my intuition again, I asked Sally if she could yell. She couldn't. She couldn't even shout. She just squeaked out tiny sounds. So, I gave her some homework: Her favorite place was the beach "Go to the beach and scream as loud as you can."

"It took two days", she said but she did it! I mean she had suppressed for years how she felt, not saying the things she wanted to say, and this had made it impossible to shout. Sally healed from her surgery in record time. She got her voice back because I invited her to trust herself, to be honest about what she wanted, and to follow her own intuition.

We all need to be heard. And sometimes we are looking for permission and need to be asked what we want, just to remind us that we know. As mind/body pioneer Louise Hay said,

> *"You have the power to heal your life, and you need to know that. We think so often that we are helpless, but we're not. We always have the power of our minds...Claim and consciously use your power."*

Life can be overwhelming. Add in a cancer in our bodies or a traumatic birth experience and it's easy to lose touch with that power, especially when the experts are giving you advice that you know is wrong.

We're not crazy to trust our inner voice. And sometimes it takes extreme challenges to remind us how important it is to regain this ally. Welcome to Superpower Number One, connecting with that higher intelligence and harnessing that power.

Activating Superpower #1 - Life

Become the master of your emotional state.

If fatigue, stress, or negativity pay you a visit, transform your physical state to shift your perspective. Go for a refreshing walk, take off your shoes, and step outside onto a patch of grass to ground yourself, let loose with some joyful jumps, or break out your best dance moves to your favorite Jam. Just like a magician changing hats, altering your physical state can magically reshape your mindset and emotions. Channel your inner Mel Robbins and remember that controlling your focus and physiology puts the reins of your emotions in your hands.

1. Superpower of life action steps

1. Embrace gratitude: Start a daily gratitude journal to acknowledge and appreciate the blessings in your life.
2. Nurture living things: Care for a plant or a pet. Cultivate the responsibility and compassion that comes with taking care of another living being.

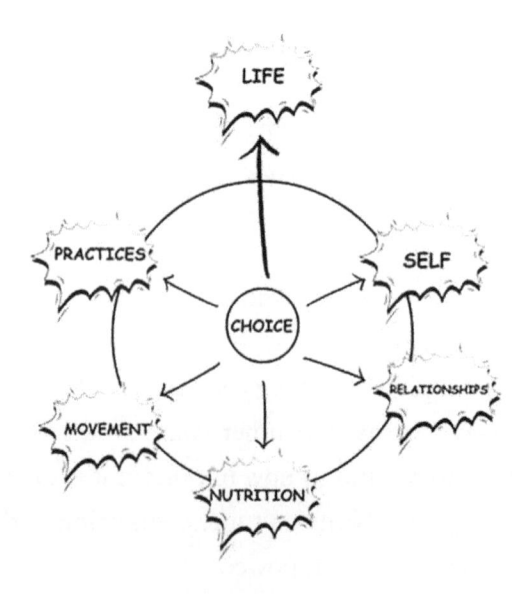

CHAPTER 2

THREE HATS ARE ENOUGH

"Stress is not what happens to us. It is our response to what happens. And response is something we can choose."

—Maureen Killoran

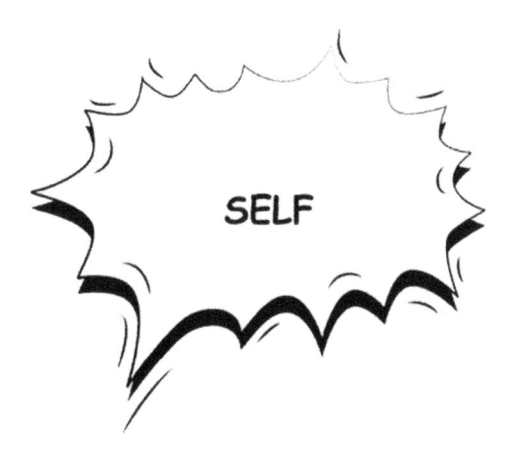

(illustration: burst shape labeled "SELF")

I was married, but I lived like a single parent. My husband was a world-renowned jockey who traveled most of the time. When he was home, he was so busy that our family time was limited. Meanwhile, Jacob was in and out of the hospital constantly. I figured out that before he was five years old the two of us had spent a total of two years and three months in the hospital together.

I also had an older son to care for. Josh was in every sport available in his school: baseball, soccer, flag football, and basketball. So – all you moms know this story well - there were the constant practices after school, long weekends driving to games, and the better he got the higher level he moved to and the more demanding the schedule became. I remember many Thanksgiving games, freezing in the pouring rain, watching Josh play soccer and screaming from the top of my lungs:

"Go Josh!!!!!!!"

Being a Mom

Like other mothers, my day started early, driving Jacob to school five days a week from age two. This meant leaving the house at 6:15am to fight traffic and arrive by 8:00am, driving with the rearview mirror reflecting my mouth so he could read my lips from the back seat as I narrated our trip all the way to his Deaf and Hard of Hearing School. I'd spend the whole day with him then rush home, grab Josh, rush him to practice, then return home to cook dinner… Oh, add in speech therapy three days a week for three years plus a business and a calling (more on these shortly), and you can begin to imagine the stress.

Stress was my middle name.

Stress? That was my middle name. I was a poster child for stress. I'm sure you mom's get it. "Mothers are the world's best jugglers: family, work, money—they seem to do it all. However, all that responsibility can often leave moms feeling overstretched and stressed out.

"According to an APA 2010 survey, women are more likely to report physical and emotional symptoms of stress than men, such as having had a headache (41% versus 30%), having felt as though they could cry (44% versus 15%), or having had an upset stomach or indigestion (32% versus 21%) in the past month. The same survey also reported that women are more likely than men to report that they eat as a way of managing stress (31% versus 21%)."[5]

Eat Healthy

Comfort food wasn't an option for me. I was under strict doctors' orders: eat healthy! That was their pronouncement when I was diagnosed with uterine cancer, six months after I'd given birth to Josh. But what did "eat healthy" mean? They didn't exactly tell me. Eat iceberg lettuce with lemon and no carbs or sugar?

Back then, that's what I thought a good diet was. And, that I couldn't eat or drink anything I liked, that I should starve myself and then exercise for an hour every day. That I couldn't go out with my friends or family to a restaurant, couldn't have Cajun food or all the other foods that I grew up eating, like gumbo, rice and gravy, red beans and rice, and jambalaya. Of course, I also believed that it was OK to eat Entenmann's Danishes because they were fat free!

Calories in, calories out!

But I learned how important healthy food was to my survival, to keep up with my hectic lifestyle and manage my own healing. I came to understand how nutrition, exercise, and mindset are all necessary for good health. Because I was forced to, I learned how to stay healthy, and this started me down the road to my career in nutritional consulting.

*Like many professionals, my calling grew
out of an urgent personal need.*

Back to the mom challenges. Of course, our duties never stop, they just move in another direction. I wasn't just a (mostly single) parent, I also had a business to run. I owned and managed a Cajun

---

[5] https://www.apa.org/topics/parenting/supermom

Food Restaurant with my brother Kevin. The business was extremely consuming. Our average workday was 7:30am to 1:00am, six days a week. Then we would spend our one day off cleaning and ordering food, doing the payroll, and scheduling workers.

But as my responsibilities with Josh and Jacob intensified, especially while my husband was on the road, it became obvious that I could no longer be a chef, cook, and manage the restaurant. It was too much. I felt guilty when the burden shifted to my brother, but he understood, God bless him. I wasn't just raising a family; I was keeping my cancer at bay.

I learned how to make a very structured plan and stick with it, because there was only one of me managing three other humans in my immediate family, two dogs, one cat, one turtle, two hamsters, an aquarium of fish, two bunnies, one pygmy goat, 23 horses, and let's not forget 17 employees.

I was wearing three hats: mom, businesswoman, and self-healer.

Finding My Calling

It's that third role that has grown into my life's calling and that's what this book is about. My personal story might be interesting but I'm only sharing these stories so you can understand what motivated me to develop my health care business and to hopefully inspire you to expand your understanding of health. We teach what we need to learn, right? I'm teaching what saved me, from the stress of a three-ring circus life and cancer in my body. Because of this background, I know firsthand that what I share with my clients works. It worked with me first. And it can work for you.

Healing myself had to become my primary task.

This introduces our second Superpower: Self. Most of us have an unconscious relationship with ourselves. We're aware of the self-talk, how we judge ourselves and react to what others say about us. But it's all reactionary. Meanwhile, we all have this amazing superpower, which some call "self-esteem."

Accessing and activating this superpower is simple but not always easy. It's about appreciating ourselves. Well, easier said than done, given that many of us grew up in families where no-one was aware of how important this is in our early maturing years. But it's never too late to begin loving ourselves. When we do, it makes it easier for others to love us. And, health-wise, having a loving attitude towards ourselves is like having a secret weapon to fight disease.

I can appreciate myself so much more now than I did back then. I was actually pretty amazing! I was actually wearing three hats, but I came to realize that I couldn't keep wearing any one of them if I didn't survive. So, I began to educate myself and dove deep into the world of personal self-care. I became an aerobics instructor, a personal trainer, a holistic nutritionist, then a life coach.

I was 40 when I finally knew what I wanted to be when I grew up.

Food is Medicine

I learned that eating itself, something we do every day and mostly unconsciously, can become a positive lifestyle practice. It's much more than physical. Healthy eating can become a way to center ourselves, a pathway to understanding who we are, what we need, even how we give and receive love.

Who are we being while we are eating?

Most of my clients show up with eating and drinking habits that come from a place of emotional restriction and deprivation. Those inner problems can't be solved with food. I help them understand that when we diet, get on the scale, and see that we lost weight, our subconscious tells us, "Good job, you can cheat now! You have some wiggle room now!"

*This will be our reward for working so hard,
we tell ourselves. We deserve it!*

Or, we stumble through a diet without ever quite getting it. Why? Because we're trying to use old habits to create new behaviors. We are forcing ourselves to abide by new rules without changing our lifestyle. We do things halfway, then get on the scale again and now it says we've gained weight, or it's stayed the same. This time our subconscious says, "I might as well throw in the towel. This stupid diet isn't working!"

Time for some ice cream!

"Over time, the associations we have with food become solidified. We celebrate birthdays with cake, we celebrate soccer game wins with pizza parties, and we make ourselves feel better after a breakup with a pint of ice cream. Because it's so commonplace, people don't take the time to think about their own eating habits such as what they eat, when they eat, and why they eat. Beyond that, people might not have a good gauge on when their eating habits are entering a danger zone."[6]

Crowding Out the Crap

Nathalie was a client who suffered from constant pain. She was a nurse, on her feet all day. Her joints hurt and she was not sleeping well. She gained weight and couldn't lose it. Nathalie ate at the hospital crapateria, as we called it. Mac n cheese soup (seriously), breakfast burritos, pizza. Hospital food does not make you well. In Nathalie mind, she was defeated before she even started.

I kept hearing the same desperation from another nurse client. She drank iced lattes throughout the day and espresso on her evening breaks. Her typical dinner was ice cream. Then, because she couldn't sleep, she needed coffee all day and was so emotional exhausted from the stress of her job that she felt hopeless.

---

[6] https://www.sbm.org/healthy-living/when-does-eating-become-a-problem

I teach my clients a profound secret:

Don't take things away, crowd them out.

We don't count their calories. We don't take out all the carbs, coffee and alcohol because socializing with their family and friends was really important. Instead, they began substituting in health foods and crowding out the unhealthy ones. Both clients very quickly improved their sleep and began to feel rested for the first time in years.

They became more positive and happier, and even better organized. They both watched the pounds melting off. They became their old selves again.

The healthy foods I recommended were also delicious, so they began to think, "Hey, I get to eat this!" rather than, "I have to eat this."

It's All in Your Mindset

We've heard the phrase, "It's all in your mind." Actually, it's all in our "mindset." I help clients stop categorizing food as good or bad and rate them instead either as food that fuels and heals their bodies or food that depletes their energy and make them sick. I introduce them to a simple formula:

Increase the good fuel, decrease the energy drainers, enjoy the benefits.

The key is to start with a healthy mindset: decide to be healthy. From that place, we can then address the imbalances in our diet and lifestyle. "What do I have too much of or too little of and what changes would restore balance?"

Getting Started

Overwhelm is the enemy; planning is our ally. In later chapters we will zero in on the many simple changes you can make, substituting healthy choices for habitual ones. But you can get started right now with what I'll call our first Healthy First Habit:

Drink enough water.

Most people are dehydrated. So, learn to drink water - not soda or coffee - throughout the day. Make this your new healthy habit #1. It's free! Begin first thing in the morning. Fill a glass with 16 oz of water, squeeze half a lemon into it, and place it on your nightstand every night. When you get out of bed, drink the entire glass before you do anything else. This is the fastest way to hydrate and flush out the toxins that your body began to expel while you were sleeping.

This is your first step. It seems so simple. But you will notice the benefits right away. As you add more healthy self-care practices, you'll quickly find a rhythm and begin to enjoy your new priority – becoming healthier. A surprising side benefit that many clients report as they advance down this road is that their feeling of self-worth increases. They watch themselves becoming a better version of themselves and that feels good.

They are activating Superpower #2 – Self.

I don't know how many hats you're wearing in your life. I was wearing three and that was overwhelming until I made a plan and prioritized self-care. And everything changed when I made my own wellbeing number one. This was not selfish for me and it won't be selfish for you. After all, we can't take care of anyone else if we're sick. Self-care really takes off when we access that second superpower: developing a loving, appreciative relationship with ourselves.

Activating Superpower #2: Self

Prioritize your self-care.

Start each day with a nourishing breakfast. Treat yourself to a healthy meal within one hour of waking up. Include protein-rich options like eggs or a delightful smoothie. Elevate your meal with antioxidant-rich fresh berries or embrace the goodness of healthy fats like avocado, nuts or seeds.

Picture this: scrumptious scrambled eggs and sliced avocado with roasted sweet potato and apple hash. Feeding your body well at the beginning of the day isn't just about sustenance; it's an act of self-love and respect that will resonate throughout your day. Eat food that will love you back.

Other Action Steps

1. Practice self-reflection: Set aside regular time for introspection, journaling, or meditation. Explore your thoughts, emotions, and write down 5 aspirations every day.
2. Identify strengths and passions and talent. Make a list. Find ways to align them with your personal and professional life.
3. Prioritize self-care: Develop and commit to a self-care plan that includes activities like exercise, mindfulness, adequate sleep, drinking water and nourishing your body with balanced meals. (example: Protein, greens, healthy fat & a carb).

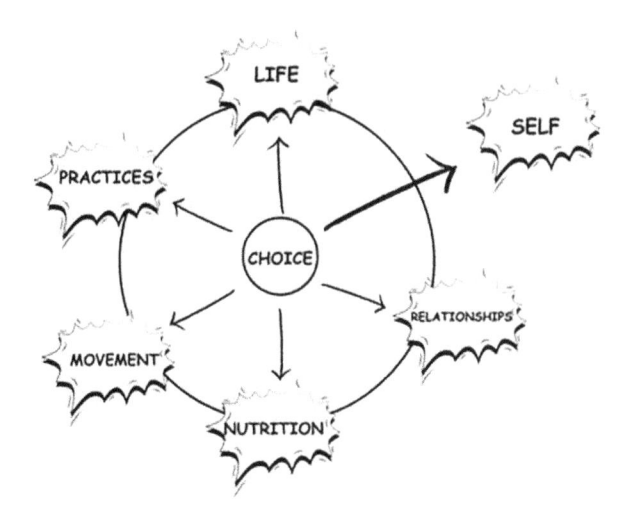

CHAPTER 3

FOUR CHINS

*"Every time you are tempted to react in the same old way,
ask if you want to be a prisoner of the past or a pioneer of the future."*

—Deepak Chopra

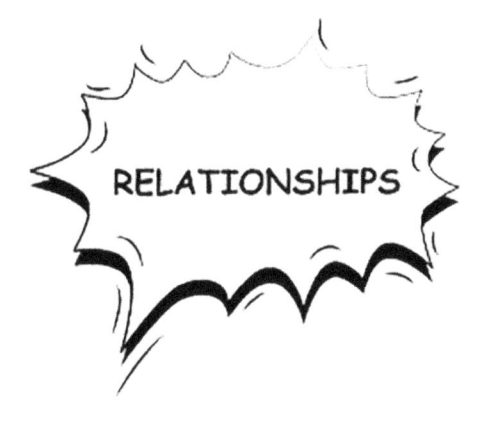

RELATIONSHIPS

"**W**e're not sure if he's going to make it," the doctor tells me. "If his brain stops bleeding, he has a chance."

I am 23 years old, pregnant, and my jockey husband of 3 years has just been crushed in a racing accident. But hearing he may die is not the only terrifying news a doctor has told me lately. I was just eight weeks along when I am issued this grim warning: "I'm sorry. Your cervix has rejected the stitches we put in to hold your baby, so your body is constantly trying to go into labor. You absolutely must remain in bed for the remainder of your pregnancy. If there's any hope for your baby to survive, you must never stand up for more than five minutes at a time."

So begins months of confinement to bed at home, while my husband is at work all day. I'm alone. I'm deathly afraid of losing my baby. I'm also dreading a phone call that tells me Kent has been injured. How dangerous is being a jockey? An ambulance follows the horses around the track.

That phone call comes, at the worst possible time.

We'd been trying to have a baby for the three years we lived in California. All my family was back in Louisiana and Texas so when I finally did get pregnant and this complication arose, I didn't really have any close friends to help me.

Life became terribly tedious.

Every day, I lay in bed watching TV, reading magazines, only getting up to go to the bathroom. My husband would make me a sandwich each morning around 6:30, put it in an igloo ice chest with water next to the bed, and leave for the track. As soon as I woke up, I'd strap a belt around my belly that was connected to a telephone relay through to the nurses station at the hospital. I'd lay totally still for an hour while this mechanism monitored my body. I did this twice a day. No one visited me. For months. And my husband often didn't get home until eight or nine at night. Those were long days.

When I needed more medication, we would leave the front door unlocked so the pharmacy delivery person could come right into the house and upstairs to leave the medicine by my bedside. I didn't see the downstairs of my home for six months.

It's December 11 around 5:00pm when the phone rings. It's one of my husband's jockey friends and he's hysterical. I can barely make out what he's saying. I finally figure out that he has been trampled by a horse in the last race and it's really bad. "You have to get to the hospital!" the friend shouts. I hang up and the phone immediately rings again. It's a doctor from the ICU: "You need to get here right now … your husband is not going to make it through the night!"

My head is burning with an instant fever. How am I going to get to the hospital? It's on the other side of town, an hour and 20 minutes away in traffic. What do I do??? The only thing I can think of is to call his agent. I ask if he can come and pick me up; he says he's already on his way but he's a long way off. I call my doctor to let him know that I'm going to the hospital. He says, "Absolutely not. It's too risky." I insist and he finally relents but demands that they first determine how many contractions I'm having. "If it's under four contractions an hour I'll let you go."

I hook up the system and lay still for a full hour. It's maddening. I can't cough, cry, or sneeze. If I do, it registers as a contraction. After an hour, the nurse calls to report. "Sonia, you're at eight contractions an hour." The doctor forbids me to go anywhere. "Well," I tell him, as the agent arrives, "I'm on my way to the hospital right now!"

I lay down in the backseat of the car. When we arrive and I step out of the car, two nurses rush up with a gurney. "Are you Sonia? Yes? Lie down! We're taking you to the ICU to see your husband."

Moments later, I'm in the room beside him. It's a moment I will never forget. He's fighting for his life, screaming in pain, his eyes are protruding, he's covered in dirt and has 16 skull fractures. His head is horribly swollen and he's bleeding from both ears; the nerves in his right ear have been severed.

I do the only thing I can do. I talk to him. I tell him how beautiful our baby is going to be. I tell him that I need him, that we both need him, that this is the start of our family together. "I can't do this alone," I cry.

They wouldn't allow me to stay so I went home. Back in bed, I made a call to my mom to let her know what was happening. She said "You'll probably go into labor pretty soon, as stressed as you are." But that would make the baby 10 weeks premature so I assured her that wouldn't be happening.

The next day I heard from the hospital. He was awake, he was talking, he was ordering people around. That's when I knew he was going to be OK. A few days later, I heard a knock at the door. It was my mom. She had flown out from Louisiana. Finally, for the first time since the accident, I felt like I could take a breath.

Moms know when their babies need them.

We settled in for the night but I woke up five hours later with a sharp pain, feeling like I had just peed. Oh no, I thought, not yet! I yelled for my mom. "I think I'm going into labor." We jumped in the car and headed straight to the doctor's office. Dr. Morrison agreed. "You're having the baby today!" (SP#3)

I made a call to hospital. They had just moved him from ICU the day before. His agent answered the phone. I told him that I was going into labor and to please let my husband know.

I've been in the hospital now for six hours and who rolls in on a gurney and stops right next to me? Yup, my husband! He checked himself out of the hospital, against doctors orders, and laid down in his agent's car's backseat just like I had only five days before. He can barely see through tiny openings around his eyes because his face is so swollen. He can't lift his head and has no idea what's going on. I'm not sure he even knows where he is. But he's here, with me!

Dr. Morrison enters the room. He takes one look at the two of us and says, "This is the saddest thing I've ever seen." I read his face and know that something's wrong. Something else. "Is it the baby?" I ask. "Please, please check on the baby."

You never want to see panic on your doctor's face.

Suddenly, orders are being shouted and nurses are literally throwing me from the bed onto a gurney. As I'm being wheeled down hall, Dr. Morrison tells me, "I'm so sorry. The baby is in distress. We must do an emergency C-section immediately."

The next thing I remember, someone is slapping my face and shouting. Someone else is shaking me. "Wake up. You've got to stay awake. Your baby needs you."

What? I see my mom and the agents wife standing over me. Nurses are running around. "You can't go to sleep," one of them tells me. "You must stay awake. If you fall asleep, you might not wake up again!"

I hear talking in the background about possibly inducing a coma. I look at my mom and ask her what's going on? She's crying. I hear one of the nurses say, "You have toxemia, preeclampsia. If you want to live to see your baby, you have to fight to stay awake. You cannot fall asleep."

Toxemia is an infection in the bloodstream that affects the nervous system, the liver, kidneys, stiffens the joints, and swells you up like crazy. It is also the second most common cause of maternal death.

Moments later a nurse arrives, holding my four-pound two ounce baby boy. Josh is alive and in the world! He is the tiniest, hairiest little baby boy I've ever seen. His head is smaller than an orange. I'm awake now! My baby needs his mom! He has fought to survive every day for the last eight months. As I battle my fatigue and pain, I feel my body begin to swell. I am filling up with fluid.

A few days later I dared close my eyes to rest when I heard, "That's not her. She's huge! She has four chins." I slowly opened my eyes to see my husband, backing out of the room in a wheelchair.

I asked the nurse for a mirror. She said, "No, you shouldn't look at yourself yet, you're a little puffy." A little puffy? I later found out that I was now 43 pounds heavier than when I arrived, at the hospital pregnant.

I eventually recovered and lost all that inflammation and weight. After learning how to heal myself, before I even knew I was using my superpowers. Josh survived and he's a healthy boy. My husband got well. We were married for 20 years when we divorced. It's taken many years to integrate all the lessons I learned from this experience.

*I now understand how strong we
can become when we have a reason to live.*

I also know how our own voice is the most important one, to hear it and honor it and do what we know we should do, like risk death by going to the hospital to see your injured husband.

Although I didn't know it at the time, this was where my holistic journey really began, a journey that has taken me into a career of helping others face their health challenges and know that they too can make it through.

I couldn't have gained the confidence I have today without those life-threatening experiences. I know firsthand the difference that our attitude makes. Doctors, technology, medicine, it's all important and I wouldn't have survived without their help. But I also know that what ultimately tipped the scale in the right direction for me, what helped me survive and deliver a healthy baby against the odds, was faith. I never gave up.

This is what I teach my clients.

The Power of Loving Relationships

When I read back over this chapter, I counted 10 relationships with people who cared about me when I needed help: my husband and his agent, the jockey friend of his, two different doctors, three nurses, my mom, and another friend. Some of them barely knew me yet they still helped.

When we are kind towards others – which is how we are all designed to be – they feel this instinctively and are happy to help us when we're in need. This highlights our third superpower, loving relationships.

Staying healthy has so many levels to it and one of them is having a support system in place when we can't take care of ourselves. My writing coach told me how friends made meals for them for a month when his wife was recovering from cancer surgery. One friend coordinated the volunteers who chose days and food would magically appear in a cooler on the front porch every day at 5pm. He told me that their generosity meant more to them than the physical food. They tell people that their friends helped to rebuild her body.

Of course, relationships are important all the time. Think of it like having a bigger body, one that contains all your family and friends. Just like you want your physical body to be healthy, it makes a difference when the larger body of your relationships are healthy too.

Sharing The Faith

Laurie came to see me because she wanted to lose weight. When I asked her what her goal for an ideal weight was, she had an exact number. I asked her when was the last time that she had weighed that and she said 17. She was 35 now.

When I asked about her debilitating fatigue, chronic joint pain, and insomnia, she didn't seem as concerned about those symptoms. As we worked together, I noticed that the only guide she used for success was the scale. She was happy when her number went down but when it didn't, she would exercise for hours, six even seven days a week.

I made a deal with her. She agreed to stop weighing herself and do a selfcare practice instead. She had removed the mirror in her bathroom and only used a compact mirror to put on make-up. So, I asked her to look in the mirror every day and say "I am beautiful. I am lovable. I am caring. I am worthy. I am healthy." I also gave her a journal to start writing down all the negative things she was telling herself.

I call them ANT's – Active Negative Thoughts.

This was our starting point and it's where I often start with clients. If you become aware of how you talk to yourself, and you are thinking negative thoughts like, "I'm fat, I'm ugly, I will never lose weight no matter what I do," you will soon realize that your body cannot heal when it's conflicted. You can eat gluten free, paleo, you can fast, exercise every day, you can take all your vitamins, but if you don't have the tools to process your life stressors and trauma then you will never become healthy. And you will never feel worthy, truly believe that you are beautiful, and you will never be fulfilled.

Laurie changed her negative talk. She began to erase her negative programming and to believe in herself. Her symptoms began to clear up. And she lost weight. Best of all, she came to realize that it was her mindset that really did it. She had to begin believing in herself. Then, all the practical physical things she did could have their full beneficial effect.

This chapter introduces superpower number three: relationships. As you read, there were many people who helped me. It's amazing how that happens, how allies show up when we need them. But we can also be proactive and adjust our relationship matrix, to spend more time with those who are positive than those who might drag us down. I picture this like the solar system; each one of us is the sun and others are like planets orbiting around us. We want some people closer than others! And some people show up like comets, streaking through our lives. Some land in our system and stick around, others keep on going and vanish into space. It's wise to know who to hold close and who to let go!

Coming from my years of traumatic experience, with my victory over life threatening conditions, I've arrived at this simple recommendation for becoming truly healthy:

Activating Superpower #3 - Relationships

Harmonize your relationships.

Nurture authentic connections by sharing a genuine compliment with someone every day. Embrace the loved ones around you, infuse positivity, and let your holistic energy create ripples of kindness. Embrace this daily ritual, and watch your relationships respond in beautiful ways.

Other Action Steps

1. Cultivate empathy: Practice active listening and seek to understand others' perspectives without judgment. Put yourself in their shoes to develop deeper connections.
2. Express appreciation: Regularly express gratitude and appreciation to the people in your life. Write heartfelt notes/emails or engage in small acts of kindness to show you care.
3. Build a supportive network: Surround yourself with positive and like-minded individuals who inspire and uplift you. Step away from relationships with those who feed off your energy but don't exchange. Join communities or groups with similar interests.

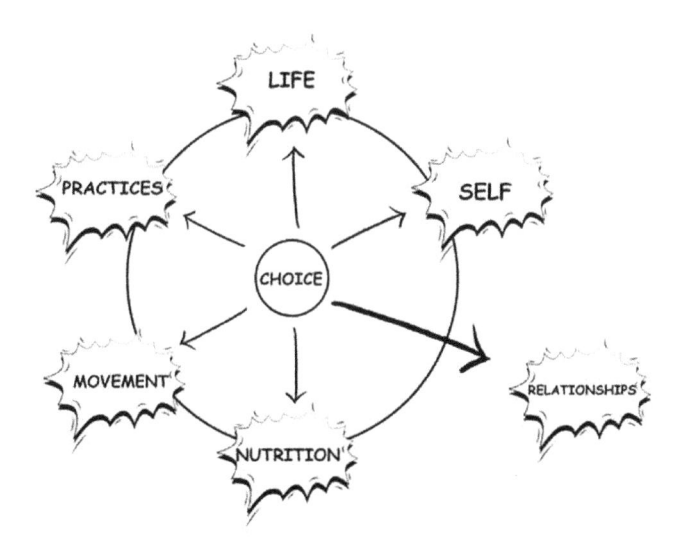

CHAPTER 4

BEAUTY REALLY IS AN INSIDE JOB

"True beauty comes from the inside out, it emerges from proper thinking as well as proper nutrition and exercise."

—David Wolfe

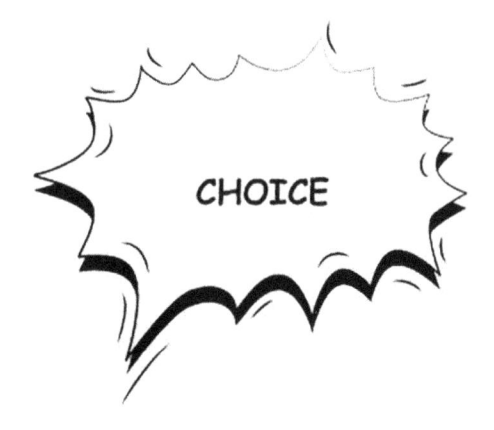

CHOICE

I actually did have four chins, and I've never felt so ugly in all my life!!!!

It was painful for me to even look in the mirror. I'm 5'3" and suddenly I was as wide as I was tall! It was difficult to walk. I would cry when I needed to get dressed to leave the house because nothing fit. The circulation in my arms was being cut off by my sleeves. My boobs were exploding the buttons on my blouse so that I had to get reinforcement Velcro sewn in between the buttons just to keep it closed!

I reminded myself every morning that I *could* get through this. That my body was filled with toxins. That I wouldn't look like this forever. My relationships with family and friends were so important and I had to work at not feeling ashamed of how I looked when we were together. But it was easy to stay on purpose and to focus on ridding my body of all the toxins because, for one thing, I knew how much my beautiful son depended on me. I was on a mission and helping myself was to lay the foundation for helping others.

Many of us struggle with concepts about beauty, even in the best of times. Those judgments can develop a running dialogue of negative self-talk. We judge ourselves, and we judge others for how we look compared to them, even though we know the concept about beauty being more than skin deep.

What image do we have of ourselves? Just how do we think we are supposed to look? Social media tells us one thing, the mirror tells us another! But we're not here to measure up to someone else's (or society's) standards of beauty.

> *True beauty comes from within, and I learned that it's spelled H.E.A.L.T.H.*

I also learned that how I feel about myself is a much better standard for beauty/health than what I look like. This noble belief really came to the test when my reflection was so abhorrent. It's a challenging concept to get but, once grasped, things really start to change, health-wise, because we all want to look our best and when we realize the role that health plays in beauty, there's an extra measure of motivation.

Changing how we measure beauty, value ourselves, and make our way into a healthier and happier way of living does start with the right attitude, but we must put the right stuff in (and on) our bodies. Mindset first, nutrients follow. We're all perfectly unique, and once we've embraced the connection between beauty and health, we can develop what I call the Healthy Body Blueprint. To provide an example of this, meet my client, Daniella.

Daniella told me that she never felt beautiful, not ever. But she *was* physically beautiful, thin, she wore elegant clothes, and had plenty of money to spend on spas and skin care products. When people told her she was beautiful she would just roll her eyes. She had a sick image of herself, and this reflected in health problems.

Daniella suffered from deeply embedded self-worth issues. Chronic pain in her joints and ligaments, debilitating Migraines, And lot's of Bloating and digestive problems. We worked together on absorption of her minerals, aiding her digestive system and lymphatic system. But what was the most challenging was how she felt about herself. I helped her learn how to heal her ANT's (Active Negative thoughts) by monitoring her self-talk. This quickly improved her mental health as she changed how she felt about herself. Soon, she started hearing comments like, "Did you change your hair… have you been spending time in the sun, because you are glowing?" Nothing physical had changed. What people were seeing was a result of the new way she was seeing herself.

Daniella *did* have a glow about her, and it was the beauty of inner health and confidence that changed how she looked.

She started radiating positive energy from the inside and this was reflected on the outside. Daniella improved both her beauty and her health, and it started with clear thinking.

Introducing The Healthy Body Blueprint Program

My program has three phases:

1. Detoxification
2. Gut healing
3. Blood sugar balancing

But don't worry, it's simple. Before we get in the details in a later chapter, we need to take three simple steps to prepare for starting this program, to gain the maximum benefits. And before that, we need to tap into superpower number four: choice.

I often think this is the most important one because choice is what makes everything happen. We can choose to stick with our routines, following our habits that make us sick, or we can choose something better. The fact is that all of us are making choices every day and most of them are unconscious. We drive the same way to work every morning, we eat the same kind of food, we watch the same TV shows.

Meanwhile, we have this superpower within us, the power to choose. Keep this in mind while you read the rest of this chapter. You'll learn so much and have the opportunity to make positive changes, but you'll *always* have to choose: the same old same old or something better, something new.

Step 1 - Forget the Numbers

For many of us, numbers hold all the power! Examples:

- The numbers in our bank account.
- A test score.
- How many calories we eat. (all calories are not created equally)
- The final score in the big game when our team is playing.

We give tremendous meaning to all kinds of numbers but there's one that reigns supreme for many of us and that's <u>the number on the scale</u>! That's not something I allow with my clients. In fact, I can't tell you how many scales I've confiscated! I once had eleven of them in my office, true story.

Most of us have a number in mind for what we believe that we "should" weigh, or – more likely - what we used to weigh back in the day. This becomes our goal, and we might believe in it, wholeheartedly.

We may place an almost supernatural significance on that number, believing that our life will be transformed when we hit it.

Forget what you weigh and what you want to weigh.

Where does that weight number actually come from? And does a number, any number (but especially this one) truly have the power to fulfill us and make us happy? How about our mindset, the way we feel about ourselves, our relationships with family and friends?

> *"The beauty of a woman is not in a facial mode, but the true beauty in a woman is reflected in her soul. It is the caring that she lovingly gives, the passion that she shows. The beauty of a woman grows with the passing years."*
>
> —Audrey Hepburn

Step 2 - Have a Beautiful Mind

One way to increase self-confidence is by practicing positive affirmations. I've recorded a guided five-minute MP3 program that lives on my YouTube channel, complete with instructions. You start with short statements like, "I am beautiful" or "I am worthy." Repeating these phrases to yourself daily can help train your brain to focus on the positive and ignore the ANT's. Feeling better about yourself also helps you manage stress, which can produce a significant health benefit.

"In <u>one small study,</u> participants who affirmed their values had "significantly lower cortisol responses to stress" compared with the control group, researchers wrote, referring to the body's primary stress hormone. <u>Another small study</u> of college students found that those who did two value-affirming writing exercises ahead of a midterm exam had lower stress levels the day before the test. Self-affirmation can also help improve problem-solving under stress, according to <u>a 2013 study</u>…

Brain studies offer further insight into how self-affirmations might work, experts said… Affirmations seem to engage regions of the brain associated with positive valuation."[7]

Placing sticky notes on your computer or bathroom mirror is also helpful. Try changing your morning routine if you brush your teeth with your right hand brush your teeth with your left, this will stop the robotic morning routine. Then before you leave the mirror, look yourself in the eye and say "I Love you" 10 times. You're training yourself to show your inner beauty to the world. So, do whatever makes you feel confident because the more you exude inner beauty, the more others will see it and be drawn to you.

> *"Nothing can dim the light from within."*
>
> —Maya Angelou

Step 3 - Clean Up Your Act

We live in an increasingly toxic world. "Every time we breathe, eat, drink, wash, exercise, get dressed, go to work or climb into bed, we expose ourselves to potentially harmful substances – <u>air pollution,</u> synthetic chemicals, contaminated food and water, radiation, pharmaceuticals, <u>alcohol,</u> noise and microorganisms, to name but a few."[8]

How serious is this? "Every year, between 9 and 12 million people die prematurely through the cumulative effect of such exposures, mainly air and water pollution, heavy metals, synthetic chemicals and workplace carcinogens and particulates."

This is a real wake up call for anyone who believed they weren't in danger because they aren't exposed to obvious toxins in their workplace and don't live in air polluted cities. Sadly, toxins are everywhere. We can't

---

[7] https://www.washingtonpost.com/wellness/2022/05/02/do-self-affirmations-work/
[8] https://www.newscientist.com/article/mg25333710-800-how-our-environment-is-making-us-sick-and-what-we-can-do-about-it/

do much about most of them, but we can learn how to take care of the ones that affect us the most personally, those right in our own homes.

When our bodies are healthy, they can excrete excess hormones, cellular waste, etc. every day. But when this waste removal system malfunctions, things get clogged up and symptoms begin to appear.

Incredibly, the average woman applies over 500 toxic ingredients to her body before she leaves the house!

During the day, we all come into contact with over 300,000 toxins.

I don't mention this to scare you. Instead, it's important health information, meant to empower you to mitigate toxin exposure so you can detoxify your body in safe and effective ways to gain optimal energy and health. But we can't start doing that before you learn what products to avoid and get them out of your life.

Here's what I consider a health law: Read the label! Here are ten of the most toxic ingredients that show up in everyday products that effect our weight, our hormone balance, and can cause disease.

BUTYLENE GLYCOL, DEA (DIETHANOLAMINE), MEA (MONOETHANOLANIINE), SODIUM LAURYL SULFATE (SLS) & (SLES), SODIUM HYDROXIDE, POLYETHYLENE GLYCOL (PEG), PARABENS (ANY PARABENS), ALCOHOL, ISOPROPYL (SD-40), MINERAL OIL, COLOR PIGMENTS, FRAGRANCES & DYES.

Obviously, we can't remember all these names (and there are thousands more). The simple rule is to avoid chemicals. Chemicals are easy to recognize, they have non-food names. And be especially aware of the term "natural ingredients." That doesn't mean it's good for you to consume, not everything that is in nature is good for you and it's usually mixed with unnatural chemicals or flavorings.

It Starts in Your Bathroom

If you can't put it in your body, don't put it on your body.

"Researchers have found dangerous levels of mercury in skin lightening and anti-aging creams; they've linked chemicals in hair dyes and straighteners to breast and uterine cancer; they've traced fragrances in soaps and shampoos to poor semen quality and fertility issues. Most American children are also exposed to toxic chemicals—from a wide variety of sources—that may be a cause of learning and developmental disorders, obesity and asthma.

"To be sure, not all chemicals are bad for your health. And you're just as likely to encounter unsafe chemicals in processed foods and drinks, home furnishings and even prescription medicines as you are in personal care products. But low doses of iffy chemicals can add up over time and with exposure to multiple products, said Dr. Shruthi Mahalingaiah, an assistant professor of environmental, reproductive and women's health at the Harvard T.H. Chan School of Public Health."[9]

In preparation for beginning the Healthy Body Blueprint Program, where we begin to detoxify your body, I'm going to ask you to detoxify your bathroom. Get a big box and start going through all your beauty products. The skin products, the hair products, the cleaners, everything. You want to get rid of everything with chemicals.

Don't worry, there are literally thousands of healthy alternatives. In fact, here's a list of options:

1. Skin care: Skincare, Body washes and Make-up
    - All-natural skincare: i.e., Annemarie Gianni Skin Care,
    - Facial moisturizer: i.e. Avalon
    - Body Washes: Avalon, Pacifica, Dr. Bronners

---

[9] https://www.nytimes.com/2023/02/15/well/live/personal-care-products-chemicals.html

- Make-up: Annmarie Gianni, Pure Minerals, Mineral Fusion, Beauty Counter, one of my favorites!
- Sunscreen: i.e., Badger, Kiss My Face, or make your own it's easier than you think.

2. Hair care: Hair Care Products
   - Shampoo: Aubrey Organics, Avalon Organics, Desert Essence
   - Conditioner: Giovanni, Intelligent Nutrients, John master's Organics

3. Cleaning products: Cleansers and Soaps
   - Facial soap or cleanser: Annemarie Gianni Skincare
   - Liquid hand soap: Pangea Organics, Hugo Naturals

This chapter introduces superpower number four: choice. As you read, there are many healthy choices you can make about what you put in and on your body. When this superpower is activated, choosing what's healthy becomes natural and automatic.

Regardless of our age and body shape, we are all essentially beautiful and can improve our beauty with the healthy choices we make every day. Let your beauty emerge from the inside! Make new choices by activating that superpower, the power of choice!

Activating Superpower #4 - Choice

Say "Yes" to whatever improves your wellbeing.

Embrace the concept of nurturing your body, mind, and soul with foods and activities that uplift your spirit. Say no to highly processed or sugar-laden treats that might momentarily tempt your taste buds but leave you feeling less than your vibrant self. Choose foods, exercise, and relationships that energize you and make you feel amazing both inside and out. Remember, the choices you make impact not only your momentary mood but also your long-term well-being. Treating your body with kindness through healthy food and activity choices is a beautiful expression of love.

Other Action Steps

1. Identify your values: Reflect on your core values and align your choices with them. Make decisions that are in line with what truly matters to you.
2. Practice mindfulness: Expand awareness of your thoughts, emotions, and reactions. Pause before making impulsive choices and consider potential consequences.
3. Embrace change: Be open to choosing new experiences and possibilities. Step out of your comfort zone and take calculated risks.

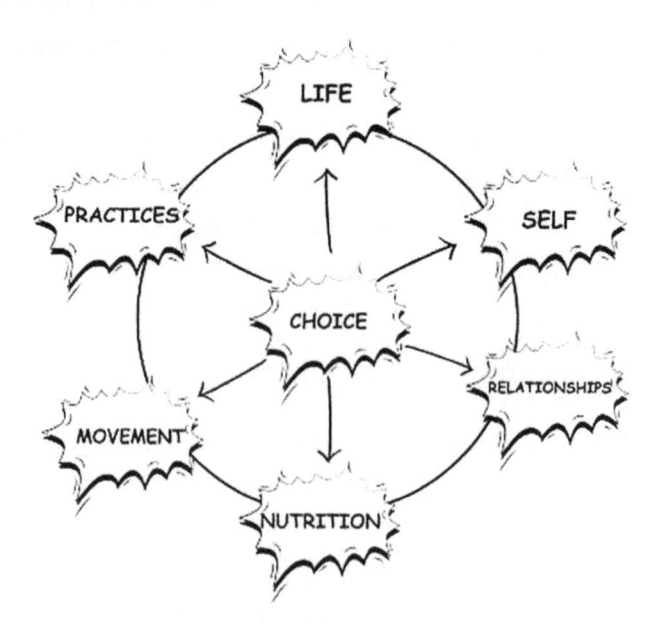

CHAPTER 5

YOU ARE MUCH MORE THAN WHAT YOU EAT

"To live is not to stay in the shallow waters of our fears of ineptitude, of our insecurity. To live is to swim into the deep; alone, but not lonely; afraid, but with courage; content with all that is, marveling at the ambiguous, miraculous wonder of being."

—Tor Syvrud

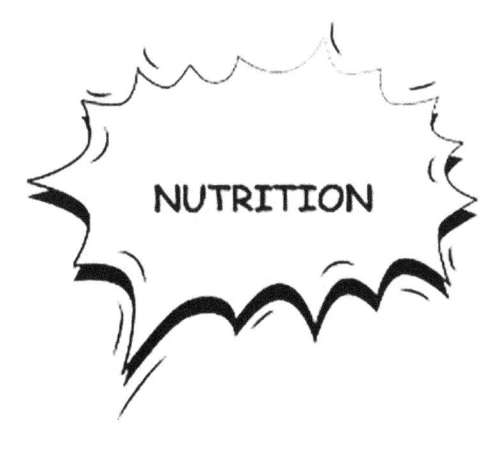

NUTRITION

"Although I didn't know it at the time, this was where my holistic journey began…"

That's what I wrote in the last chapter, having just described my nightmare experience in the hospital, almost dying during pregnancy from toxemia, having a premature baby, with my husband on his death bed from severe injuries, lying next to me.

I know that sounds bad, and it was! All 3 of us was in ICU in the same week! But just as bad was being told by doctors that what I knew was right for my own body was wrong.

Once I left the hospital and started along the road to recovery – which included losing the extra 40 pounds plus the baby weight! I'd put on - doctors told me eat less and exercise more. Really? As I told them, I was already exercising six days a week for at least an hour and a half. I was eating super healthy, or so I thought. But, month after month I looked the same (obese) and I felt the same (sick). I was still in pain, and I was not losing weight.

Finally, I got sick and tired of the doctor's looking at me as if I was secretly scarfing down cheeseburgers and French fries at every meal and being lazy when I was actually starving my body and abusing it with excessive exercise. I reached a tipping point and decided to take matters into my own hands.

*I realized that if I wanted to get a different result,
I would have to **do** something different.*

This was the official beginning, the birth moment of my commitment to wellness, to take full personal responsibility and do whatever it took to regain my own health and help others do the same. It all started with that realization and a simple but profound commitment to honor the wisdom in my own body. And this is exactly what I would teach others.

My Life's Work Begins

Joshua is six months old when I go in for a personal checkup a couple of weeks later and that afternoon, I get a call. "Sonia, please come into the office first thing tomorrow morning; the doctor needs to talk with you." I'm exhausted because I was up all-night with Josh, who was not feeling well. Hmm, I wonder, what could he want to talk to me about?

He gets right to the point: "Sonia," he tells me, "You have Endometrial Uterine Cancer."

What? It can't be! What is he talking about? I'm 24 years old. Haven't I gone through enough? I ask, "What does this mean ... what are my options?" He begins to talk about a hysterectomy and external beam radiation therapy in combo with chemotherapy. "You need to speak with an oncologist," he continues. "Also, talk with your family to decide what to do."

I'm crushed. I've believed that I'm on the road to recovery. Well, it turns out that my body is full of toxins. In fact, my entire system is inflamed. But I'm still breast feeding, and I want more kids. There has to be another way. I've begun following holistic practitioners who have healed their patients from cancer, diabetes, heart disease etc. And, NO, absolutely not, I'm not going to tell my family. I know they would never agree with any decision other than these invasive procedures. I'll only tell my husband; I decide on the car ride home.

I meet with the oncologist, but I have a plan. I tell him, "I'm going to try nutrition, a functional medicine approach, immune system support, and detoxifying my body." You can imagine his face and what he was thinking of all this!

"You don't understand," he tells me. "We need to surgically remove your womb, your cervix, and your ovaries.

"Well, maybe," I reply. "But first, I want to continue breastfeeding my baby and I want to have another baby. I need some time."

My "awakening" has just gone to another level. I realize that if I want to physically survive, I will need to stay on my healing path... forever. The health of my body needs to become and remain my top priority. And health, I realize, is entirely personal, a different process for everyone. This turns out to be the most important lesson I'd ever learned and becomes the core principle in my new career.

Now my research began in earnest. I was searching for answers, reading about whole food, cellular recovery and repair, detoxification, how to have proper cellular turnover, how to assimilate nutrition, how vitamins and minerals penetrate on a cellular level, etc. I became obsessed with learning about the science of healing through nutrition and, even more importantly, attitude.

I started my recovery protocol with The Budwig protocol and food that is now called G-BOMBS, all the microgreens, wheat grass, and barley grass I could find. Vitamin IV's, Immune therapy, Infrared light therapy, salt baths, oxygen therapy… I didn't let up! And, 22 months later, I went back to see that same doctor.

> "I don't understand," he said. "Your biopsy shows that you're in remission. I don't know what happened. This makes no sense!"

30 years later, I'm still cancer free and I never had any of those procedures. But I'm always aware that the cancer could return at any time, so I have to practice what I preach. And my research never ended. I now have eight degrees in Holistic Nutrition and Wellness counseling and am constantly adding to my education. I have a robust practice with clients who share my healthy obsession with healing. I know that I'll be doing this work for the rest of my life.

> "The point is not to live longer but to live better, not just to add more years to your life but to add more life to your years."
>
> —Dr. Mark Hyman

You Are What You Eat (and much more). So, Don't Be Cheap, Fast, or Convenient

Nutrition is our fifth superpower. When I say nutrition, I'm including everything we put into our body, including liquids, plus everything we put *on* our bodies, like lotions and sprays. What guides our choices? Think about how food is advertised. What sells us? Price and taste and appearances. Nutrition? Not even an after though.

Imagine opening a menu in a restaurant and reading about the specific nutritional value of what's offered. Some restaurants use codes for Gluten Free (GF) and Dairy Free (DF) and Organic (O). What if there was much more detail? For instance, this cilantro salad can help to cleanse your liver. Wouldn't that be something?

"You are what you eat" is such a profound statement, but I'd heard that for years without caring what I was putting in my mouth and how it might be impacting my health. Why was that? Something was getting in the way of acting on what I knew. I discovered a profound way to solve this disconnect through working with a client named Mary.

Mary was a bad ass boss, in charge of over 100 managers, excelling at a highly stressful job, but way beyond overload every day. In the midst of all this, she felt alone and disconnected from everything and everyone. Getting home late every day, she would fix a quick meal for her family, which included two young adult children and older parents she was caring for. All this left little time for Mary. So, she resorted to more quick fixes for herself: over the counter medication, entertaining distractions, fast-food lunches at work, etc.

Her problems were obvious, and she desperately wanted to change. So, why couldn't she? What was getting in the way? It didn't take long to discover that Mary needed more than better time management and a good diet. Why had she created such a challenging lifestyle? So, one day I asked her a simple question I would come to use with all my clients:

"Who are you being when you are eating?"

It was quite a moment.

This question led us toward the heart of things. Mary was unhealthy. She was unhappy. In fact, she had a whole lot of "un's" going on. She felt unseen, unheard, unattractive, unappreciated, and—most importantly—unloved. And she was trying to fill those "un's" with toxic food. Her food felt like it was the only thing that brought her JOY????

Who was Mary being when she was eating? An unloved, unhealthy, unhappy victim.

I created a model to help her and other clients understand what I call The Un Spiral. Regardless of which one is most dominant for any person—and there are many "un's" besides those that I just listed—I discovered that they all tend to lead to one deep core feeling that everyone who was physically unhealthy seemed to have: the feeling of being unloved.

Here's the truth as I've learned it working now with hundreds of clients:

> *Until a person puts their health first, they can circle around forever feeling unhappy, unattractive, unappreciated, and unloved without really knowing how to do anything about it.*

But they can also choose a different path. I call this coming to a "Choice Point," where they decide to face how they are feeling, go all the way to the center, and face their feeling of being unloved.

Actually, there are two choice points. The first is the commitment to becoming healthy, facing the "un's," whatever they are, and confronting the feeling of being unloved. The second choice point is deciding to love yourself. This initiates your journey back out along the same spiral but this time you find yourself shedding those "un's," arriving back at a new starting point, ready to be healthy.

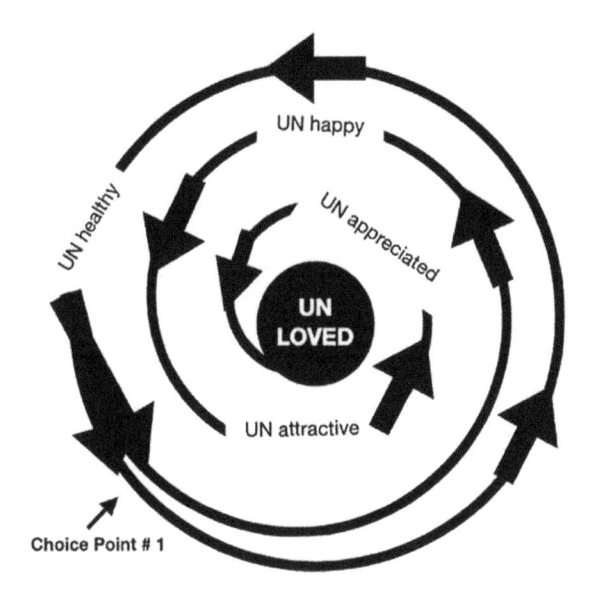

Figure: Downward spiral with UN happy, UN healthy, UN appreciated, UN attractive circling UN LOVED. Choice Point #1 indicated.

The truly magical realization that comes from all this is that the conscious recognition of feeling unloved seems to initiate the process of positive change. If we do feel unloved, at some level, why not be the one to change that… by loving ourselves first! And what better way to show this then with self-care.

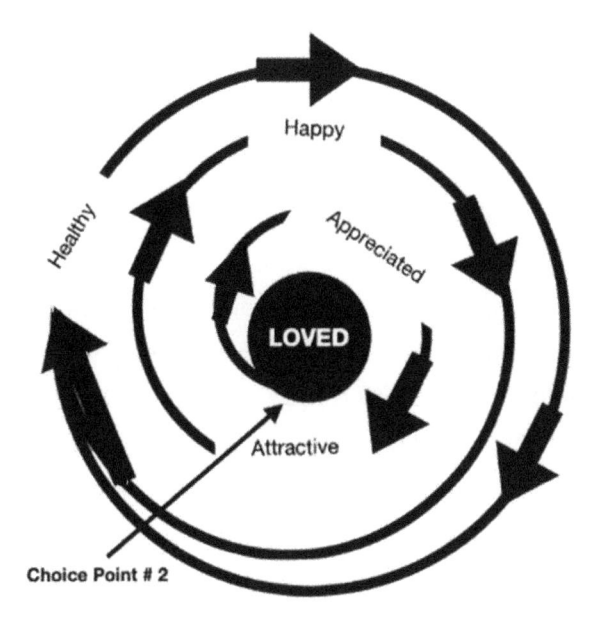

Figure: Upward spiral with Happy, Healthy, Appreciated, Attractive circling LOVED. Choice Point #2 indicated.

You *Can* Get There from Here

I came up with four priorities to guide clients who acknowledge their unloved self and decide to get healthy. This grew out of my own personal experience when this became a matter of life and death. What I developed combines inner awareness with outer actions.

You Matter

Once a person decides they are worthy of love and commits to becoming healthy, they also commit to "quality." They won't any longer just shovel something convenient into their bodies. They understand that if they really are what they eat, then only the best organic foods, non-GMO, etc. is appropriate fuel for them. With that commitment made, it's just a matter of researching how to find which superior nutrients are ideal for them and developing an affordable plan for eating well.

Be Aware

We learn to take time to eat and not eat while multitasking.
Here's what I tell clients:

If you're eating, eat.

Every time you put something in your mouth, you're either promoting health or promoting disease. Sit down and take the time to enjoy what you're eating. Be thankful you're able to give your body the nourishment it craves. Chew your food well. Some doctors advise that each bite should be chewed 30 times.
Try counting and you'll be shocked, as I was when I first explored this idea. Most of us don't chew more than seven or eight times before swallowing. So, slowing down - maybe we can get up to a dozen, or even 20. Chewing helps with digestion and prevents us from over-eating so

we won't feel bloated, We eat less but feel more nourished. And, when we take more time over meals, we are more likely to be consciously aware and grateful for what we are blessed to receive.

Be in Nature

Reconnecting with the natural world reminds us that we are part of the circle of life. Go outside and spend at least 20 minutes a day in nature. This helps us slow down to the speed of life. We get the Vitamin D our bodies need especially standing in the morning sun and, even more important, we can regain our sense of belonging in the natural world. Try taking your shoes off and standing on the grass, to ground your body first thing in the morning. You'll get the sense of deep belonging that only nature can give us to settle our soul.

Drink Enough Water

Our bodies are about two thirds water. But the vast majority of us are chronically dehydrated. This causes fatigue and memory loss, it interferes with immune response, and it can cause kidney stones, etc.

There's a simple formula for making sure you drink enough healthy water every day: Divide your weight by two and that's how many ounces you need every day. For instance, someone who weighs 120 pounds should be drinking 60 ounces, about six 10-ounce glasses, every day. That's shocking, right? If you keep track for a day or two you will be surprised. BTW, coffee, black tea and sodas don't count! For better absorption of water and to remove excess water retention try a pinch of Celtic Sea Salt on your tongue in the morning wait for it to dissolve then drink about 4 ounces of water. This practice will change how your body absorbs and let's go of water. This will support the kidneys. Celtic sea salt has 82 minerals our body needs. (This is not white table salt).

Mindfulness Assignment

Give yourself a memorable experience of these four priorities:

1. Recognize that you are worthy of love and make a commitment to love yourself by choosing to become healthy.
2. Practice conscious eating, taking time to really enjoy your meals.
3. Spend some time in nature, with no agenda except to feel that you belong.
4. Drink enough water for a day or two and see how that feels.

Simple, right? But… will you, do it? Breaking inertia to create new, healthier habits, is always the hardest part. I believe in you!

Activating Superpower #5 - Nutrition

Nourish your body with vibrant, nutrient-rich foods every day.

We first eat with our eyes so delight in the rainbow of colors on your plate – from crisp greens to juicy reds – and savor the energy and vitality they infuse into your being. With each mindful bite, chew your food well to ensure proper digestion to fuel your body and your unstoppable spirit.

Other Action Steps

1. Nourish your body: Adopt a balanced and nutritious diet that suits your unique needs. Focus on incorporating whole foods, fruits, vegetables, and lean proteins.
2. Explore new flavors: Experiment with different cuisines and recipes. Try new ingredients and cooking techniques to enhance your culinary skills and expand your palate.

3. Mindful eating: Practice mindful eating by slowing down to chew well and to savor each bite, paying attention to your body's hunger and fullness cues, and investing in a healthy relationship with food.

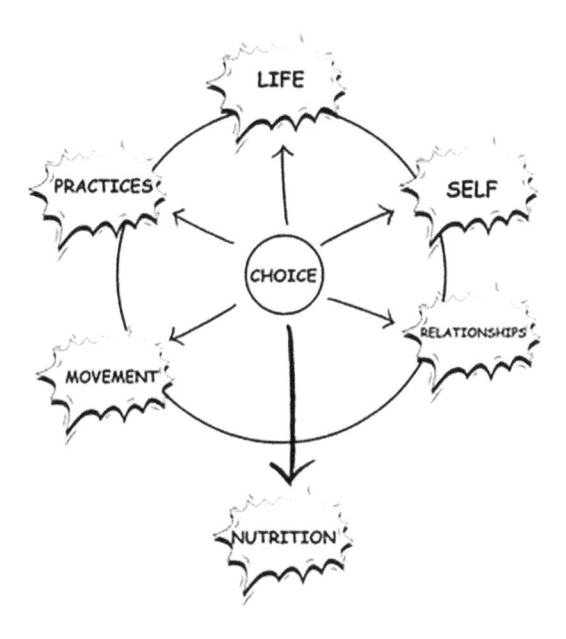

CHAPTER 6

MOVE IT OR LOSE IT

"All is a miracle, so smile, breathe, and go slowly. Walk as if you were kissing the earth with your feet. Drink your tea slowly and reverently, as if it is the axis on which the earth revolves."

—Thich Nhat Hanh

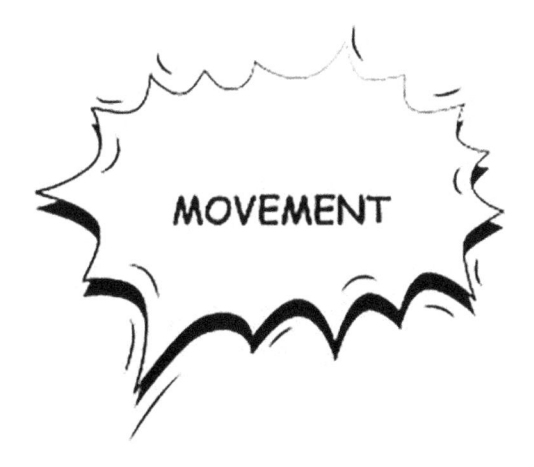

MOVEMENT

Thich Nhat Hanh pioneered the mindfulness movement, which has inspired millions of us to pay more attention to where we are in the moment. We've learned to use our senses to tune in and align ourselves with our surroundings, to be and move in harmony with other life forms. This is a vital aspect of holistic health.

Movement is a natural aspect of life. Blood moves through our bodies, impulses flow from our brains, through our nervous system.

When movement slows inappropriately, stagnation occurs. The same is true in nature. Moving water stays fresh, still water becomes an unhealthy breeding ground.

An underlying health principle here is that "movement is change." We tend to think of change as something special, something that occurs now and then, like changing jobs, trying a new diet, moving, etc. But change is constant and so, ideally, is movement.

> *"Movement is a medicine for creating change in a person's physical, emotional, and mental states."*
>
> —Carol Welch

By bringing conscious awareness to our bodies in the present movement, we deepen our connection with ourselves and the world around us. Mindful movement practices such as yoga, Tai chi, Or Qigong, and blended breath, all foster a profound sense of tranquility and inner peace.

Becoming more conscious and proactive about movement can help us develop a harmonious lifestyle that increases wellbeing and longevity. Through experience, we come to understand the interconnection of all aspects of movement within the body that generate and sustain balance. Daily movement also helps us maintain the best possible mindset, not only through physical exercise but movement in our mental and emotional aspects, as well as our spiritual growth.

The irony of movement is that we also deepen our experience of stillness. It's like being in the eye of a storm, with movement all around yet where we are everything is calm.

This describes the "witness" state, long held to be the ultimate evolved state of consciousness. But, just because we feel increasingly still within, doesn't mean that we shouldn't move our bodies! In fact, we *need* to move them to keep them flexible and healthy. This is something that is also being acknowledged psychologically. In fact, some mental health professionals are now prescribing exercise for relieving depression.

> *"Movement is the song of the body."*
>
> —Vanda Scaravelli

"Several randomized controlled trials have supported the efficacy of exercise interventions to alleviate symptoms of mild-to-moderate depression to a degree comparable to other evidence-based treatments, including medications and cognitive behavior therapy."[10]

> *Movement can be as healing as drugs or therapy.*

What's Best For You?

Each person's body is unique, with distinct strengths and limitations. To discover the best movements for you, we need to understand our body's diversity. Embracing body diversity means honoring and celebrating our bodies just as they are, identifying our individual capabilities, and being compassionate with ourselves during our journey to ultimate health. Even then, we avoid getting stuck in habitual routines. We listen to our bodies, adjusting our movements to suit our needs and avoiding activities that may cause harm. We also avoid adopting one-size-fits-all fitness goals, By respecting our body's wisdom, we cultivate a sustainable and lifelong relationship with daily movement.

Functional fitness is a core aspect of holistic daily movement, focusing on exercises that improve our ability to perform everyday task with ease and efficiency. Functional movements mimic real life activities, such as lifting, carrying, or bending, to enhance our overall function and reduce the risk of injury. By incorporating functional exercises into

---

[10] https://www.ncbi.nlm.nih.gov/pmc/articles/PMC4545504/

our daily routine, we align our fitness goals with the practicalities of daily life, enriching our holistic health journey, improving our quality of life, and increasing happiness.

> *"True enjoyment comes from activity of the mind and exercise of the body; the two are ever united."*
>
> —Wilhelm Von Humboldt

Movement Keeps Us Young

Regular exercise actually helps us feel younger by slowing the aging process. Erica Eller, in her blog Science-Backed Reasons Why Exercise Makes You Younger, shares these specifics:

Increases energy efficiency

Makes our skin younger

Improves posture

Improves flexibility

Boosts mental capacity

Keeps our metabolism high

Slows cell aging

Relieves stress

Lowers cancer risk[11]

Regular movement sustains "energy efficiency" which means that, as we age, we will maintain our ability to continue moving around easily.

---

[11] https://healthyhumanlife.com/blogs/news/exercise-makes-you-younger

Exercise increases blood flow, nourishing our skin cells by sending them more oxygen and carrying away the waste. Sweating is healthy because it purges toxins that would otherwise clog up the system.

As we age, we experience muscle loss and bone density diminishes which affects our posture. We've all seen elderly people stooped over… that can be a sign of many problems but it's likely an indicator of lack of movement over many years. Seniors especially are advised to develop a regular workout routine that utilizes resistance bands or weights. Swimming is ideal, as is walking, sometimes referred to as the best exercise of all.

Yoga and Pilates are excellent practices for maintaining our flexibility. If you haven't done this type of exercise, you might find it challenging at first but it's worth hanging in there until you begin to enjoy the results. Once you experience the renewal of your body – which can happen to some degree at any age – you'll quickly adopt these as regular practices. You might have avoided yoga because you are physically inflexible. Well, isn't that the best reason to begin doing it?

*When you are more flexible, you decrease
your risk of injury and increase your longevity.*

Aerobic exercise affects our brains, promoting the healthy growth of brains cells, growing new blood vessels, and increasing the size of our hippocampus which is responsible for memory and learning. This means that we can maintain a young brain as we age, to continue learning. What a great investment in quality of life during our elder years!

And what about maintaining our ideal weight? Aging means that our metabolism slows down and pounds can add on, which means we are at a higher risk for diabetes, heart disease, etc. Maintaining muscle mass means that we burn calories efficiently (which keeps our weight down) to reduce the risk of serious illness.

Exercise helps us look, feel, and actually *be* younger because it literally turns off the aging process in our chromosomes, keeping our

DNA healthy. The caps at the end of our chromosomes are called telomeres and they get shorter as we get older. Exercise can actually lengthen them, slowing aging and extending our life span.

Then there's stress. Stress itself can be healthy. We stress our muscles when we exercise them. If done properly, that's good. But what's unhealthy is how we react to stress, if it produces anxiety. We need to learn how to bounce back from adversity. Here's where meditation is useful and even more so, walking meditations in nature.

Finally, to quote directly from Eller's work (I was paraphrasing above):

"Some studies suggest that regular, moderate exercise may reduce the risk of <u>some cancers.</u> One study showed that regular physical activity can reduce the risk for colon cancer in men by about 24 percent. Other studies show that regular exercise may reduce the risk of lung cancer by up to 20 percent. Plus, once diagnosed, exercise may help keep cancer from spreading."[12]

Movement Practices

Here are a few movement practices that I teach my clients. *Nurturing in Nature*

To be truly well, it is vital to embrace the healing power of nature. Make sure you are incorporating enough outdoor activities, such as walking and hiking, forest bathing, swimming, grounding or gardening. Develop a deep and intimate connection with the natural world because this promotes mental clarity, emotional resilience, and provides spiritual nourishment. Spending time in nature reminds us of our interconnectedness with all living beings, grounding us in the present moment and supporting our holistic, well-being.

Fostering Playful Creativity

---

[12] https://healthyhumanlife.com/blogs/news/exercise-makes-you-younger

Daily movement practices need not be restricted to structured exercises. They can also encompass playful and creative movement. Dancing, art, spontaneous movement, even freestyle workouts can unlock our creative potential, inviting spontaneity and joy into our lives. Embracing our playful nature fosters a positive mindset, encouraging us to approach daily movement with enthusiasm and excitement, infusing our practices with lightness and pleasure, nurturing our holistic health on a deeper level.

Cultivating our Mind Body Connection

The mind body connection resides at the heart of all physical movement. Engaging in practices that integrate breath, movement, and mindfulness, such as Pilates, HIIT or Barre exercises fosters a profound awareness of our body's sensations, alignment, and energy flow. By developing a strong mind body connection, we enhance proprioception, reduce stress, and improve overall movement efficiency, unlocking our innate potential for ultimate health. Movement also keeps our consciousness fluid, normalizing change as our natural state of being.

> *"Consciousness is only possible through change; change is only possible through movement."*
>
> —Aldous Huxley

Rest and Recovery

While daily movement is essential for holistic health, so too is the practice of rest and recovery. Overexertion can lead to physical and mental fatigue, undermining the benefits of our movement practice. It is possible to get too much exercise, which can be very harmful because it creates imbalance. Healthy movement does not require hours of cardio or strength training every day. Just 20 to 30 minutes a day is truly all that we need and my clients achieve the best results when they stay consistent with this approach.

Commit to regular movement practices that involve body, mind, and spirit. Cultivate mindfulness, develop functional fitness, forge a deep nature connection, be playful and creative, and grow your mind body connection.

Embracing restorative practices, such as meditation, gentle stretch, or mindful walks, allows our bodies to rejuvenate and recover as well as sustaining our holistic health journey over the long term. Balancing movement with rest and recovery, we create a sustainable and harmonious lifestyle that supports our quest for ultimate health and being well.

With every movement, with every step we take, we deepen our understanding of ourselves and our place in the world. Exercise can be a tremendous boon to our spiritual growth. As Taraneh Erfan King says in their blog: "If you are avoiding attending to your fitness (the condition of being fit and physically well) or do not include exercise as a regular part of your life, you are missing a major link in your ability to fully access your spiritual dimension, to live joyfully and to offer your best to the world."[13]

We called this chapter Move it or Lose It to introduce superpower number six which is movement. Stagnation in the body creates a breeding ground for disease. So, you might want to consider this mantra and experiment with adopting it in your daily routine:

Activating Superpower #6 - Movement

Move it or lose it!

Dedicate time every day to engage in a physical activity that makes your spirit soar. Whether it's a brisk walk, a dance, a heart-pounding

---

[13] https://www.mindonspirit.com/blog/2020/11/15/why-is-fitness-critical-for-the-spiritual

workout, or engaging your body to thrive in motion. Embrace the empowering rhythm of your own strength and vitality as you conquer each day with unwavering energy and grace. Movement is your daily ritual of empowerment – own it!

Other Action Steps

1. Find joy in movement: Discover physical activities that bring you joy and make you feel energized. It could be dancing, hiking, yoga, or any form of exercise that resonates with you.
2. Incorporate movement breaks: Integrate short bursts of movement throughout your day, especially if you have a sedentary lifestyle. Take walks, stretch, or do quick chair exercises to boost your energy.
3. Set fitness goals: Set realistic fitness goals and create a plan to achieve them. Track your progress and celebrate milestones along the way.

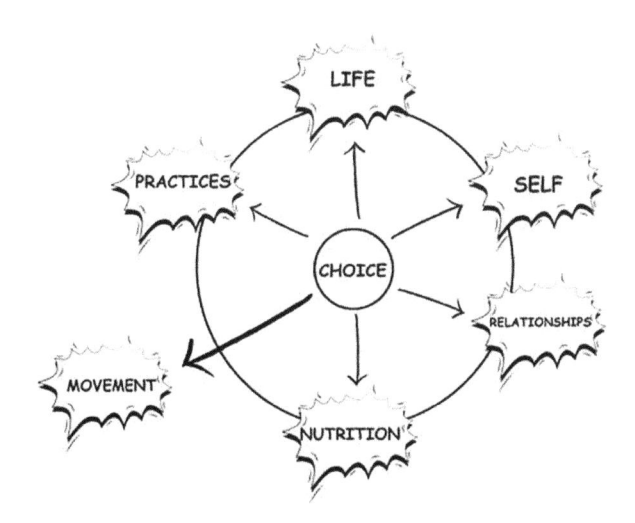

CHAPTER 7

HOW TO MANAGE OUR CRAVINGS

"Eating healthy food fills your body with energy and nutrients. Imagine your cells smiling back at you and saying: "Thank you!"

—Karen Salmansohn

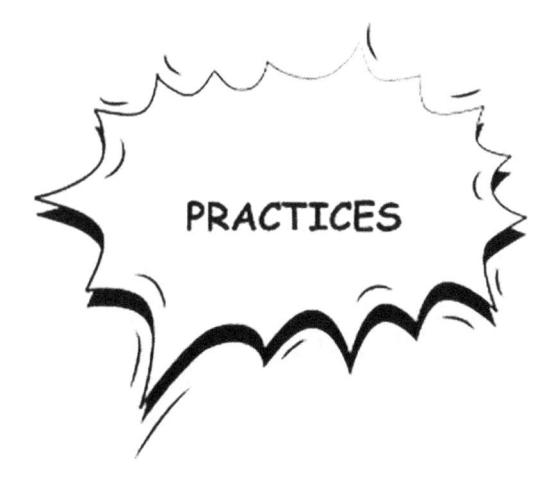

PRACTICES

Congratulations!

You've made an extraordinary commitment to your health and wellness which is proven by the fact that you're still reading here in chapter seven! Now we have a professional relationship and I'll be addressing you as if you're in my office, with one profound difference: you are what I will refer to as a "client-by-book."

I suggest that we work together over the next three months. Of course, it's obviously up to you how long you choose to take to read the rest of this book and follow through on the program specifics I'm offering. Three months would mean reading one chapter a week. The chapters aren't long and the practices I recommend are easy.

Since we'll be working together to achieve your health goals, let's start with you writing down what they are so you can commit to acting on the guidance I offer. If you email this to me at sonia@sonia-marie.com, I'll include you in an every-other-month zoom consultation.

BTW, I have plenty of additional resources for you and am available for private consultations if you need extra personal support. My website is www.soniamarienutrition.com

What is your number one health concern and what result do you want to achieve?

_____

_____

_____

_____

_____

_____

_____

_____

_____

How long have you had this condition, what is the feeling associated with your first memory of it, and what feeling could you imagine having when this heals, in one word?

_____

_____

_____

_____

_____

_____

_____

_____

_____

That feeling is now your wellness compass. Circle your word. Remember it while you read and practice; it will motivate you to keep going, especially when you encounter resistance, which *will* happen. Please read and sign the following agreement:

I am committed to full spectrum wellness in body, mind, heart, and spirit. With this commitment I give my word to:

- *Read every week and complete all the worksheets.*
- *Be open minded as I read.*
- *Be receptive to trying new foods, concepts and exercises.*
- *Fulfill the commitments I make to myself.*
- *Eat nourishing foods according to the guidance in this book.*

- *Exercise according to the guidance in this book.*
- *Pause and play and spend time in nature every week.*
- *Give gratitude for the relationships in my life.*
- *Develop a listening to my body's wants and needs*
- *Face the primary stressors in my life and manage them with the practices in this book.*
- *Finish reading the book*

Date: _____ Signed: _____

Your email address _____

Name: _____

What Are Cravings?

Having established what primary foods are in the last chapter, we can now begin a thorough study of secondary foods (the ones that show up on our plate). This has to begin with exploring a much-misunderstood human experience: cravings.

According to Harvard Public Health online, "About 678,000 Americans die each year from chronic food illness. That toll is higher than all our combat deaths in every war in American history—combined. That's right: there are more deaths each year from our food than all the combat deaths from the Revolutionary War through the wars in Afghanistan and Iraq."[14] In that same article, they report that "the economic cost of nutrition-related chronic diseases has been estimated at $16 trillion over the period from 2011 to 2020."

We know that junk food is hard to resist and that it contributes significantly to chronic illnesses. But we may not know that there's

---

[14] Jerald Mande, March 1, 2023, https://harvardpublichealth.org/nutrition/processed-foods-make-us-sick-its-time-for-government-action/

a robust industry called "food design" where scientists experiment to come up with formulas for food irresistibility.

In his book, e End of Overeating, David A. Kessler quotes Howard Moskowitz who is an expert on consumer behavior. He spoke at a recent conference about the highly competitive world of food design where the payoff is "food people want to buy (and can't stop themselves from eating)." He said, "If you can find that optimal point in a set of ingredients you may be well on your way to converting that array of chemicals and physical substrates into a successful product."[15]

In other words, foods that are bad for us that we crave.

Most people demonize their cravings. Indeed, many cravings lead to unhealthy eating habits that may become addictive, sometimes a direct result of the engineered junk food irresistibility Moskowitz spoke of. But some cravings actually give you valuable information about what's going on inside your body. It's always trying to show/tell you what it needs through various signs and one of them is what we call "cravings." e question is, what exactly is that desire for something (right now!) really communicating to you?

Here's the short take: If you are craving salty foods, it's possible you are deficient in Magnesium, Calcium, and/or Vitamin A. If you want sweet foods, you might need Magnesium (it shows up everywhere) and/or Iron.

You're craving crunchy foods? You might need more zinc, calcium, or iron. And Magnesium. Creamy foods are beckoning you? Seek out foods rich in Omega 3, Folate, Vitamin B- 12,Vitamin D, and C, and, yet again, Magnesium

I'm sure you've noticed the common thread here:

All nutritional deficiencies start with magnesium.

---

[15] Dr. David Kessler, The End of Overeating, Rodale Books, 2010, page 109

That's because Magnesium is what your body needs to absorb *every* vitamin and mineral. When you give your body the Magnesium it requires, it can do its job and keep you healthy.

Barb's Story

When Barb came to me she was completely lost. She had tried weight watchers, Jenny Craig, Keto, Paleo, the Nutria System, you name it she had done it. "I've been on some kind of diet for over 40 years," she told me with tears in her eyes. "I have diabetes, high blood pressure, high cholesterol, chronic pain in my joints and I crave sugar constantly!"

Barb could not stop eating sugar. "Sugar is my downfall," she cried. "I crave sugar all day long. Cookies, candy, cake, anything sweet. I've tried and tried and tried. And I certainly can't give up chocolate!"

I told Barb, "You don't have to."

Why was she craving sugar? Her body was desperately trying to tell Barb that she had a deficiency that needed to be supplemented. Of course, the more she ate sugar the more deficient she became. To stop the craving, she would have to take care of the deficiency.

Her body wanted chocolate, but I believed that it was actually screaming for antioxidants. Barb was deficient in, you guessed it, Magnesium.

Today, the average adult American consumes over 70g of sugar daily. That's 5.6 tablespoons a day, 10.5 cups per month and, on average, 66 pounds a year. Our children consume an average of 72 pounds of sugar per year, since most have built up a significant tolerance. This all means that when someone is *not* eating sweet foods or not eating at all, the cravings will kick in.

Sugar cravings are eerily similar to drug addiction. Some drugs cause immediate health issues and can be deadly. Sugar, on the other hand, damages the body slowly. When the body can't create enough insulin to keep up with too much sugar in the blood, that excess creates chronic inflammation and turns into abdominal fat. Too much sugar also contributes to other health problems like acne, mood swings, and accelerated aging.

> *Over the years, excess sugar becomes a catalyst for deadly conditions like heart disease, diabetes, and even cancer.*

Tens of thousands of years ago, humans used sweetness to determine which foods were safe to eat. As the centuries passed, sweet foods became more accessible and more powerful, raising the dopamine levels in the brain quickly and dramatically. Dopamine works like a reward, a pleasure neurotransmitter for the brain. When our bodies are out of balance and we are subject to our cravings, we'll eat whatever gives us the biggest, quickest dopamine hit. That's spelled s.u.g.a.r.

Crowding Out

I told Barb, "I'm not going to take your chocolate away from you. We're going to lean into your craving. I'm going to show you how to be a detective, how to listen to your body. If you are craving chocolate, then your body needs Magnesium. So, we're going to add more Magnesium rich foods into your diet. And, BTW, one of them is chocolate! ere's 65 mg of Magnesium in just one square of 70-85% dark chocolate!"

I introduced Barb to the principle of "crowding out" unhealthy foods by adding in healthy foods. Like leafy greens, avocado, banana, kiwi, broccoli, potatoes, dark chocolate and almonds, all naturally abundant in Magnesium. I assured her that before too long her cravings would change and she would want these foods, because her body would be getting what it *really* wanted.

In Kessler's book, he wrote about how healthy habits take over. "Over time, the act of eating highly rewarding food creates an automatic response. We build "action schemata," mental imprints of the actions we take and the specific sequence in which we take them. Action schemata develop more quickly and become stronger when the stimulus driving our behavior is reinforcing."[16] This explains why I asked you to identify a positive feeling you'll have when you've achieved your first health goals; that fun emotion can be a great motivator.

It's late afternoon. You're tired, cranky, hungry, and about to abuse yourself with junk food you know is bad for your health. You realize this and slow down. You interrupt the impulsive reach for what you want that you know you should not have. You pause for just five seconds and tune in to your body.

What is it saying? Does it want primary or secondary food, and what kind? Every time you do this, you change the circuits in your brain, replacing an old habit pattern with a new one. And, you improve your intuition. And now, with a measure of distance from the craving, you are free to make a healthier choice.

The Habit Loop

Dr. Kessler developed this simple model that describes what I've come to call The Habit Loop.

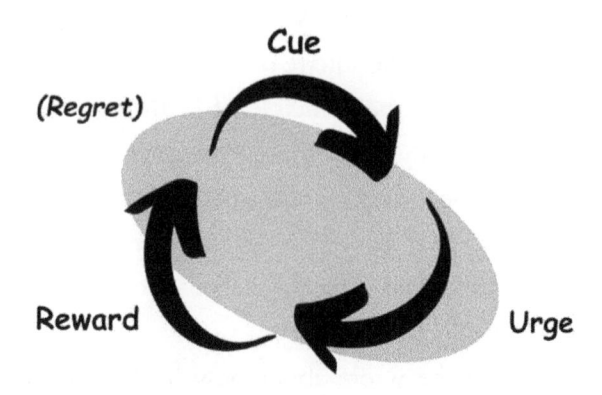

---

[16] Dr. David Kessler, The End of Overeating, Rodale Books, 2010, page 61

Our brains employ a *cue-urge-reward (regret) cycle* for survival. Kessler's model is not the only one to describe this natural progression. Authors Charles Duhigg and Nir Eyal are credited with another one, below.

In both cases we can see how this works.

1. Something cues a craving.
2. We respond in some way.
3. We get a reward.

Step three is the critical point. How do we respond? Depending on our choice, the reward will be healthy or not and we will feel satisfied or regretful.

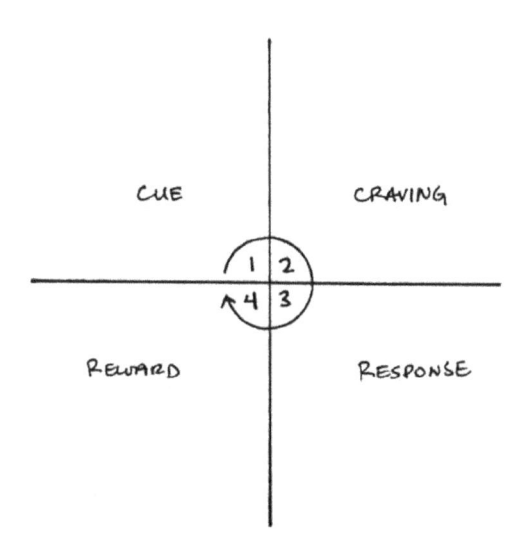

```
           CUE          |        CRAVING
                     ( 1 | 2 )
   ──────────────────( 4 | 3 )──────────────────
                     (   |   )
         REWARD        |        RESPONSE
```

"Crowding out" is about substituting healthy foods for unhealthy foods (and healthy habits for unhealthy ones). We generally break down cravings into four categories and the table below gives you a great list of healthy alternatives, organized according to which of the four cravings you have.

CRUNCHY

- apples
- frozen grapes
- rice cakes
- light popcorn or plain popcorn: use coconut oil to pop in a covered pan
- one or two hard pretzels, the large Bavarian variety
- carrots: particularly the super-sweet, organic baby carrots
- crunchy crudités of veggies and dip (hummus, tabouli, vinaigrette, favorite dressing)
- celery and peanut butter (use non-hydrogenated peanut butter)
- hummus with whole grain toast, baby carrots, rice crackers
- nuts

SWEET

- wheatgrass
- fresh, whole fruit
- organic yogurt and ripe fruit
- apples and almond butter
- sprouted date bread with jam
- frozen yogurt: freeze yogurt and make your own!
- dried fruit
- use leftover grains to make sweet porridge: drizzle maple syrup and sprinkle cinnamon, add soymilk and bananas, heat with fruit juice, etc.
- smoothies: mix whatever you have in the kitchen – fruit, ice, soymilk, yogurt, carob powder, etc.
- fruit "ice cream": peel a banana, freeze, blend in a food processor with nuts, berries or raisins and serve; can be put through the screen of a juicer for a creamier consistency.

- freshly squeezed fruit juices: Make your own and try different combos.
- sweet vegetables: yams, sweet potatoes, squashes (acorn, butternut, kabocha) cut into chunks or fries; sprinkle with cinnamon and bake.
- dates stuffed with almond butter or other nut butter
- organic dark chocolate chips or carob chips

SALTY

- olives
- pickles and pickled vegetables, such as carrot, daikon, beets and lotus root
- tabouli, hummus
- oysters and sardines
- steamed vegetables with tamari/shoyu or umeboshi vinegar
- tortilla chips and salsa or guacamole: try whole grain chips such as "Garden of Eatin" brand and freshly made salsa or guacamole.
- sauerkraut: it will also knock your sweet craving right out!
- fresh lime or lemon juice as seasonings or in beverage
- salted edamame
- small amount of organic cheese

CREAMY

- smoothies
- yogurt
- avocados
- rice pudding
- dips and spreads, like hummus and baba ghanoush

- puréed soups
- puddings made with silken tofu, avocado or mashed banana
- mashed sweet potatoes
- coconut milk

This Healthy Snack list is reproduced as a downloadable pdf file on my website. It's a wonderful print out to paste on your fridge as a daily reminder of healthy alternatives you can use to crowd out old habit non-foods.

Jacob's Story

My youngest son Jacob has a very rare disease called Usher Syndrome, specifically Ush 1c. It causes profound deafness and a balance disorder at birth, then blindness later in life. is usually starts early in adulthood with night blindness, then the peripheral vision goes, then blindness comes. In fact, Jacob now today is considered to be legally blind. It turns out that Usher has two genetic protein mutations in the same gene. He got one from me and one from his father. is is extremely rare!

As you can imagine, the remaining senses Jacob has are extra sensitive. And, he has great intuition. Because of his rare disease, he also has a lot of food texture and taste issues. Picky eater doesn't even come close!

Jacob has learned how to listen to his body and course correct as his needs change. He had to take a stand early in life, trust himself, and stay proactive with his secondary food choices. No matter what life throws at Jacob, no matter how traumatic it is I know he always puts his primary foods first, then makes the best nutritional choices when he can. He enjoys every bite and so do I because we often cook and eat together.

Jacob's resiliency and strength inspire me every day. I know this is cliched to say but if Jacob can do it, so can you and everybody else!

Rehearsing the Future

Your seventh superpower is Healthy Practices. This includes anything you do that improves or sustains your wellbeing– physically, mentally, emotionally, spiritually, and in your relationships. So, we could say that everything in this book is about the seventh superpower. It activates when we develop a healthy mindset and begin to assess everything on the basis of this question: "Is this healthy for me or not?"

I'd like to you imagine yourself adopting this mindset, changing your habits, regaining your health, and being vibrantly alive and happy, all in the near future. And imagine how you will feel. Pick one word. Like "euphoric," "peaceful," etc.

Now, I'd like you to write yourself a letter to yourself from this future moment. I'll give you an example, below, so you have something to follow. Write your own (feel free to innovate), date it approximately when you imagine having almost completed reading this book), sign it, put it in an envelope and mail it to yourself. When you receive it, store it in a safe place, and wait until the last chapter when I ask you to open and read it. Make sure to write your own customized letter. This one is just offered to stimulate your thinking. The idea is to give yourself a future reward that you know is coming… because you wrote the letter yourself!

May 5, 2024 (today's date plus the time you'll take to read the book)

> Dear (your name),
>
> This is your future self, reaching out to congratulate you. You did it! You followed through on your commitment to Sonia's healing with your 7 superpower by reading the whole book, doing all the exercises, and putting what you've learned into practice. Well done!

In Chapter Seven Sonia invited you to imagine what you would feel like in your healthy future. Remember the feeling you identified, if you can. Are you feeling it now? Or, what *are* you feeling?

You *are* healthier now. You will continue to get healthier, every day, month, and year. You will become an increasingly credible beacon of inspiration for family and friends. Imagine the many positive repercussions from what you have done.

Give yourself a big hug and a pat on the back and accept Sonia's appreciation for giving her the best reward any teacher can ever get: one more person who has followed through on what they learned from her and are sharing the wealth with others.

Good job!

Love,

(your signature)

Stamp and address your letter and put a note on the envelope with the date you want to mail it. This is a reminder of when to mail the letter. Place your letter somewhere it won't get lost and when that day comes, pop it into the mail. Also, put a tickler in your calendar.

This is the final chapter in Part One and here is the last of your seven healing superpowers. You'll find more details on my website, www.soniamarienutrition.com.

Activating Superpower #7 - Practice

Develop and practice healthy habits.

Wake up each morning and embrace the excitement of a brand-new day! Remind yourself, "Today I get to make this the Very Best day!" By repeating this affirmation, you're setting your mind on a positive track, ready to face any challenges with a smile. Remember, the subconscious mind is a powerful ally that brings your intentions to life. Even the smallest positive thought can create a ripple effect of greatness. This Practice will help you believe in yourself, and your day will reflect that belief. There are so many more practices, found throughout the book, and others you will develop.

More Practices

1. Create a morning routine: Start your day off with intention by designing a morning routine that aligns with your goals and values. Incorporate practices such as meditation, journaling, affirmations, or exercise to set a positive tone for the rest of your day.
2. Implement a regular mindfulness practice: Set aside dedicated time each day to cultivate mindfulness. This can be through formal meditation, mindful breathing exercises, or even integrating mindfulness into everyday activities like eating, walking, or washing dishes. Practice being fully present in the moment and observing your thoughts and sensations without judgment.
3. Explore personal growth practices: Continuously seek opportunities for personal growth and development. Engage in practices such as reading personal development books, attending workshops or seminars, seeking out mentors or coaches, or participating in online courses. Embrace a growth mindset and commit to lifelong learning and self-improvement.

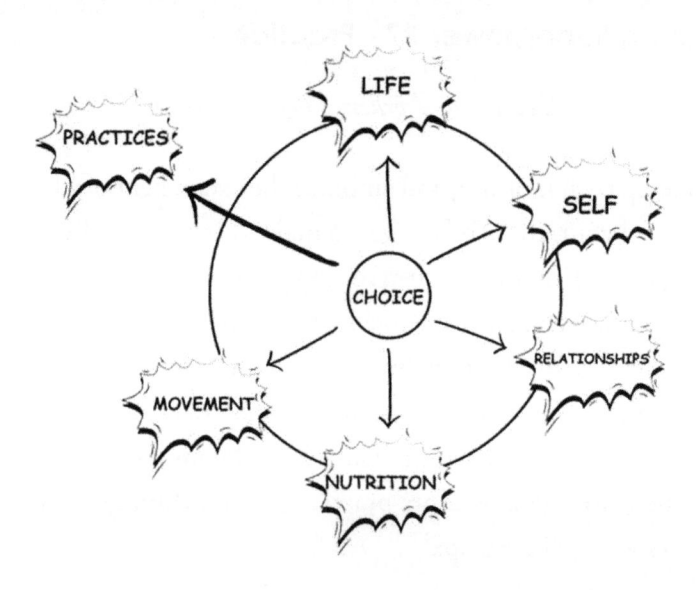

Reference: ReNue and The Whole journey, The national library of Medicine

PART TWO

BECOMING HEALTHY

CHAPTER 8

TRUST YOUR INTUITION

When you understand the connection between what you eat, why you eat, and how you feel, you will be on your way to enjoying a happier, healthier, more energetic life, with healthy cravings and no emotional eating.

—Me

Every day everywhere, millions of women and men are searching for a magical diet, the silver bullet cure for gaining energy, relieving pain, and especially losing weight, given that almost a third of all adult Americans are now overweight and two of every five of us are officially obese.

Incredibly, early in 2023, *this* actually happened: "Dr. Fatima Cody Stanford, a doctor specializing in obesity medicine at Mass General Health in Boston, claims diet and exercise have little impact on the disease that affects nearly half of all Americans, so what does she think people should do about it? "The number one cause of obesity is genetics," Stanford told CBS' Lesley Stahl.[17] Dr. Stanford is now a White House official.

---

[17] https://www.foxnews.com/media/biden-admin-expert-claims-obesity-cannot-treated-exercise-good-diet

Doctors immediately pushed back vigorously, as did just about every common-sense person who has either experienced for themselves or watched family members or friends gain or lose weight by taking or not taking personal initiative. Do genetics play a role? Absolutely. But are they the primary driver of obesity? Absolutely not. Real statistics and centuries of experience say no.

Perhaps not coincidentally, "… the U.S. Food and Drug Administration (recently) approved Wegovy (semaglutide) injection (2.4 mg once weekly) for chronic weight management in adults with obesity."[18] Yes, this drug does cause weight loss. But up to 30% of that loss is in muscle and ligaments, not really what you want to be losing. And, if you dare, read about the side effects. Yikes!

Who Are You Being While You Are Eating?

I mentioned this question in the last chapter, the one where I explain how I invite my clients to adopt a healthy mindset. Now we're diving deeper.

The fact is that while millions of health minded people *are* losing weight, regardless of their genetics, weight loss alone may not significantly improve health, even though "slim" and "healthy" are usually matched without question.

Health is not a diet, it is, first, an understanding.

Being healthy is knowing how to listen to your body and giving it what it truly needs. It's a gut knowing, an intuitive feeling in the pit of your belly, signaling your brain that something is too much or too little, not needed at all, or that you need something different. This, as you'll remember, is tapping into superpower number one: the intelligence of

---

[18] https://www.fda.gov/news-events/press-announcements/fda-approves-new-drug-treatment-chronic-weight-management-first-2014

life itself. Life is managing everything that's going on in our bodies without our conscious help. Where we *can* help is by learning to listen, to trust our intuition and make choices (superpower number four) that contribute towards improving our health.

Losing weight is a healthy side effect of developing that knowing.

This is the first teaching tool I use with clients, helping them become health detectives while they are eating, instead of food addicts, oblivious to the connection between what's going into their mouths and what stares back at them from the mirror.

Who are you when you are eating? Someone who cares about the health of their body? Or someone driven by unconscious compulsions, stress, perhaps an emotionally toxic environment? If that's what's guides *your* food choices, you're listening to the wrong voices. If you would like a daily MP3 of affirmations tune in here:

Now, we've just identified a great secret, which is also the starting point for my work with clients: how we feel often determines what we choose to eat. So, let's pay attention to our emotions.

Our Primary Food Doesn't Come on a Plate

Surprise: nutrition is our secondary source of nutrition.

I know. That's puzzling. I'm accustomed to blank stares from clients when I offer this as a statement of fact. So, I'll tell you what I tell them, to help identify what I call primary food:

- The first time you fell in love. Everything was exciting. Colors were vivid. You were floating on air. And, you probably forgot about food (unless you were on a dinner date). You were high on life.

- Being deeply involved in an exciting project. where you felt confident and stimulated? Time seemed to stop, didn't it? The outside world just faded away. And, you probably forgot to eat.
- Being a child again, playing outside with friends. Dinner time rolls around so mom call out to you. "Come in now, it's dinner time," she cries. What happens? You pretend you don't hear her! Or, you plead, "No, please Mommy, we're not hungry yet. Can we play a little longer?" If she manages to herd you inside, you probably force down the mom-approved minimum as quickly as possible, then rush out to play again.

These experiences are all primary foods... they are emotional!

On the other hand, recall a time when you were depressed, when your self-esteem was low. We've all watched movie scenes where someone lays in bed gorging themselves on chocolates after a breakup. It doesn't really help because they're actually starving for primary food – which is emotional - and no amount of secondary food (not even chocolate!) will lift their spirits, at least not more than the time it takes before the sugar high wears off.

When we feel lousy or lonely we can eat as much as we want of anything we crave but never feel deeply satisfied.

It can even be the same when we're feeling good. We come home at night, we peer into the refrigerator searching for something to eat, but what we really need is a big hug or just someone to talk to.

Primary food feeds our hearts. Secondary foods feed our bodies. And here's the key understanding to this relationship: there's no guarantee that what goes into the mouth will do much good. We don't digest food well when we're upset. So, step one for improving health (and losing weight): filling our emotional needs.

We access our primary foods through the first three superpowers: life, self, and relationships, all of which contribute to our emotional wellbeing.

The more primary food we receive, the less dependent we will be on secondary foods and the more our physical health will improve.

References: Primary Foods: IIN Joshua Rosenthal

Why This Works

It's scientifically proven that releasing endorphins and oxytocin creates dramatic health benefits. When we engage in fun activities and experience pleasure, our bodies are flooded with endorphins that enhance immune function, lower blood pressure, and improve our response to stressful events. So, give someone a hug every day!

Conversely, a decrease in endorphin and oxytocin levels increases our circulating levels of cortisol, the stress hormone that drives the fight-or-flight response. Since many of us are living under stressful conditions that cause cortisol to become chronically elevated, we want plenty of those beneficial chemicals that reduce cortisol levels.

This is a straightforward, easy to understand relationship but whoever learns about it? A regular supply of primary food is essential for sustaining good health and losing weight. But, ignorant of that fact, we fill ourselves with secondary foods and, failing to achieve the health improvements we want, become even more stressed and emotionally distressed, making us even *more* deficient in primary food nutrients. What a vicious circle!

BTW, this explains why every spiritual tradition encourages people to fast from food now and then. Deliberately reducing our intake of secondary foods enhances our appreciation for primary foods.

Creating Your Primary Food Menu

Becky was a client who couldn't tell me what kind of foods she liked. When I asked her what she did for fun, she just stared at me blankly. "I don't do anything for fun," she mumbled. "I haven't had fun in ages."

When I asked what kind of hobbies, she enjoyed she shrugged her shoulders and I noticed tears forming in her eyes.

Becky was lost. She was disconnected from joy, starving for primary foods. She had been doing, doing, doing to survive for so long, just getting through each day for years. She was a working mom with three kids who had been taught that a responsible adult worked hard and didn't waste time and money on vacations. What mattered was providing for her family. Period.

I helped Becky turn her health (and her life around) by identifying what I call "the five anchors." These refer to the primary foods that she needed but wasn't getting. I invite you to create your own anchors right now. Begin by listing those activities that bring you joy.

Write down what you love to do and experience. For instance, nature walks with friends, bubble baths, pedicures, playing with your kids, a massage, a cup of tea, intimacy with your partner, watching movies, playing tennis, listening to podcasts, reading in bed, learning a new language, etc. Record them below, then write down how many hours a week you spend in each of those activities.

ACTIVITY HOURS

_____

_____

_____

_____

_____

_____

Study your list. It may be quite revealing. How much time are you spending each week doing the things you love? At a glance, you'll be able to tell how deficient you are in primary foods. Now that you're warmed up, let's dig deeper to create your five anchors.

Make a list of your five senses, write down something that stimulates each one, then anchor one activity to each sense. For instance, if you love the sound of birds, make that the ring tone on your phone. If you love looking at the ocean, choose the best picture for your screen saver, perhaps from a beautiful vacation experience. Do this with all five senses.

SENSE ACTIVITY ANCHOR

Sight_____

Sound_____

Smell_____

Touch_____

Taste_____

Every time you see, touch, hear, smell, or taste one of these anchors, you will connect with a truthful realization: "These are my primary foods! I love these ... and I want more!" No problem. You just identified a whole menu of activities in the first list, a wide range of personally appealing primary foods.

Now, make a formal commitment to eat them. Promise to give your heart and body the nutrients they need for health and happiness. This means that, from this day forward, whenever hunger strikes, you will ask yourself: "Am I making the healthiest choice for myself in this moment?" Instantly, you'll be able to tell when you're about to make a choice that's *not* in alignment with the vow you've just taken.

This new habit will help you get in touch with what you are actually craving… and it's often not food! This takes us right back to how we started this chapter, learning how to listen to your body and giving it what it truly needs.

Congratulations. You just assumed responsibility for your own personal health by prioritizing primary foods. In the next chapter, we begin to focus on secondary foods so you can develop the physical food plan that is best for you. It won't be a cookie cutter diet off some expert's shelf; it will be totally customized for you, by you. And you'll be asking, every step of the way:

"Am I making the healthiest choice for myself in this moment?"

Adapted from Joshua Rosenthal, founder and director of Institute for Integrative Nutrition

CHAPTER 9

THE SELF CARE MINDSET

"If I could live my life over again, I would devote it to proving that germs seek their natural habitat— diseased tissues—rather than causing disease."

—Rudolf Virchow, father of the germ theory, around 1900

It's January 2. You step on the scale after the long holiday festivities. Oh, oh. You've put on even more pounds than last year. But the new year has just begun so it's obviously time for that by now familiar New Year's Resolution. This is the year, you tell yourself, the year of eating healthy, exercising more, and drinking less. You jump in with both feet, embracing what I call the Go, Set, Ready approach.

You sign up for a series of Pilates classes and start going three times a week. But after a week or two, life gets in the way and you only make it once that week. Life gets even busier. By the end of February, you've stopped going all together.

Does this sound familiar?

For many of us, it sounds a little *too* familiar. We want to get healthier, but doing the work to *get* healthier is hard. Why? Why should it be so hard to do something that delivers so many positive benefits?

> *Habits of behavior are important, but habits*
> *of thinking… that's where to start!*

According to David Marks, in his course, The Psychology of Eating, we are all made up of different character types or "archetypes." We are more than one person; we are more like a community with many players. I love the way David teaches these archetypes. He is what he explains so beautifully below. One of you might be a teacher; another is a best friend, a shopper, an explorer, a bitch, maybe a rebel!

Let's explore a few of these. So, The Rebel. She's the explorer, an eternal teenager always testing the limits, breaking the rules, and proud of it! She is brave, courageous enough to stand up for what's right, and forges a path forward.

How about The Perfectionist? He just has to get it right, which might lead to micro-managing. He may be a people pleaser, which could sabotage getting what he needs for himself. He could act out when told he can't have a second dessert! That's a childish response but, guess what, he or she still lives within us… it's just another role we play.

Maybe, as a child, we were told that we had to eat everything on our plate before we could leave the table to go out and play. But every child wants to enjoy the moment. And suddenly we can't, until… This is how food becomes a punishment, and how we begin to feel guilty about eating. This mindset carries over from our childhood but, as adults, we can eat whatever we want… so we do! That child in the adult body is now going to get what it didn't get back then, the freedom to enjoy. Eating the foods we crave becomes a reward. This is emotional eating, and it happens whenever our child character is in control.

> *Imagine you're on a bus and the seats are filled with all our*
> *characters. Who's driving? Let the responsible adult character drive!*

When you wrote that letter to yourself from the future in the last chapter, you had to assume a different identity. We could describe that identity or role as the "Care Giver." In this chapter, we'll explore the incredible difference that this mindset makes for your health.

The Great Debate

The Care Giver mindset is based on the idea that you can help yourself to stay healthy; you can contribute to your own healing. This belief arises from a single firm, undeniable observation: the body heals itself. While this is obviously true, as anyone who has cut themselves and witnessed the wound healing over time knows, it is not a mindset that figures prominently in modern mainstream medical care. That seems incredible, but this explains why.

"Traditional Western medicine teaches and practices the doctrines of French chemist Louis Pasteur (1822-1895). Pasteur's main theory is known as the **Germ Theory Of Disease**. It claims that fixed species of microbes from an external source invade the body and are the first cause of infectious disease. The concept of specific, unchanging types of bacteria causing specific diseases became officially accepted as the foundation of allopathic Western medicine and microbiology in late 19th century Europe. ... it was adopted by America's medical/industrial complex ... This cartel became organized around the American Medical Association, formed by drug interests ... Controlled by pharmaceutical companies, the complex has become a trillion-dollar-a-year business."

But, Pasteur's contemporary, Antoine Béchamp, proved an entirely different process, known as the Terrain Theory Of Disease. Béchamp "attained so many achievements that it took eight pages of a scientific journal to list them when he died." Here's what he presented and proved conclusively:

"We do not catch diseases. We build them. We have to eat, drink, think, and feel them into existence. We work hard at developing our diseases. We must work just as hard at restoring health. The presence of germs does not constitute the presence of a disease. Bacteria are scavengers of nature...they reduce dead tissue to its smallest element. Germs or bacteria have no influence, whatsoever, on live cells. Germs or microbes flourish as scavengers at the site of disease. They are just living on the unprocessed metabolic waste and diseased, malnourished, nonresistant tissue in the first place. They are not the cause of the disease, any more than flies and maggots cause garbage. Flies, maggots, and rats do not cause garbage but rather feed on it. Mosquitoes do not cause a pond to become stagnant! You always see firemen at burning buildings, but that doesn't mean they caused the fire..."[19]

Irrationally, we seem to care more about the quality of what we fuel our cars with than our bodies! This explains why. So, when you adopt the Care Giver mindset and begin to improve your health, you are bucking the mainstream.

You are aligning yourself with what actually works to improve health, developing and sustaining a healthy terrain in your body.

How Can We Help Ourselves?

Because we've been misled and lived our entire lives believing something fundamentally untrue about our bodies – that they were under attack from the outside and it didn't matter what we put on the inside - our relationship with food is often unhealthy. We eat, not to give our bodies what they need, but obeying emotional responses. Then we make excuses.

- "I'm too busy, I don't have time to eat healthy."
- "I'm too tired."
- "I don't know how to eat healthy; diets are so confusing."

---

[19] http://www.laleva.org/eng/2004/05/louis_pasteur_vs_antoine_bchamp_and_the_germ_th eory_of_disease_causation_1.html

- "It's too expensive. I can't afford to feed my family healthy food."
- "I don't want to eat the same, bland food every day."

Let's change this narrative. Let's learn a healthier way, one that's also enjoyable! Here are a few key facts to consider as we learn what food actually does in our bodies, which explains why food choices are so critical to our wellbeing.

- Food creates energy. Food/energy is necessary for the body to function. Every cell requires energy, and the source is from food.
- Food communicates within the digestive system, assists with metabolic processes, and aids in cell signaling.
- Foods can increase and decrease inflammation, foods can raise and lower blood sugar.
- Super Foods are essential for longevity.
- Cravings indicate mineral deficiency and/or hormonal imbalance.

Here are four factors to become aware of, to more fully understand the problems we are dealing with as we learn how to become healthier and live a long and vibrant life.

1. ***Inflammation*** is the foundation for disease. Our body directs nutrients to any inflamed area, triggering the body to redirect all signals to that injured area in an attempt to heal. Excess inflammation develops symptoms like arthritis, heart disease, cancer, diabetes, high blood pressure, insulin resistance, etc.
2. ***Hormones.*** Eating too many sugary, processed, microwaved food, too much gluten and dairy and poor-quality proteins, packaged in plastic, contributes to hormonal imbalance.

3. ***Metabolism.*** As the decades pass, your body must adjust calorie intake, according to energy output, or you will pack on the pounds. When we eat the right balance of macro and micronutrients, we have less cravings.
4. ***Detoxification.*** This is the single most important health concept to understand. We must learn how to naturally detoxify our bodies every day. Our number one fat burning organ in our body is our liver so having a clean liver is essential for losing weight.

We've Got to Move

Remember superpower number six, movement? Sickness is stagnation. All four of the above are affected by that condition. The easiest remedy for stagnation is movement. Of course, we immediately think about exercise and obviously regular exercise is essential for health. But movement is actually different. Many of us in civilized society have become sedentary. We sit all day long. We get out of bed and sit at the table to eat breakfast. We sit in our car on the way to work. Then we sit at a desk. On it goes. So, we have to be deliberate about moving and build in movement breaks. It's as essential as eating well.

Let's Begin at the Beginning

You've probably heard this before, but digestion really does begin in the mouth. Your saliva contains enzymes that start to break down starches in food as you chew. Plus, the act of chewing also signals your brain that the process of digestion is beginning. Chewing well and eating slowly gives your body plenty of time to register that you're full which means you are less likely to overeat. Chewing… the simplest movement of all!

"Maintaining good oral hygiene and oral health is an important way to stay healthy overall — not just because you feel better and look better with healthy teeth, but also because your dental health is intricately tied to the health of other systems in your body. Severe gum disease, for example, is known to cause problems in the rest of your body, including severe infection, problems with underlying conditions, and an increased risk of certain conditions associated with old age."[20]

Operating from the Caregiver mindset, your first practical step is to be in that identity as you eat. Take time for every meal, sit down and be fully present with your plate, noticing and appreciating what's on it. Eat first with your eyes, then your mouth. Don't eat in front of your computer or TV, eat without distractions. Do not eat when you are stressed because your food will not digest properly. Instead, pause a moment. Take a breath or two. Then, savor each bite and count, yes, count how many times you chew. Try for 20 to 30 times before swallowing. You will fill up faster, plus you are giving your gut assistance by beginning the digestion process in your mouth.

Sit quietly at the end of your meal and give thanks for your food.

Most of us cannot imagine life without brushing and flossing our teeth every day. But brushing is a relatively new habit, since the nylon bristle toothbrush didn't become part of our normal American experience until the late 1930's.

Our ancestors didn't brush their teeth. They didn't have toothpaste or floss for thousands of years. Yet, as archeological evidence suggests, most people throughout history lived until a ripe old age with most of their teeth healthy and intact.

Why didn't their teeth rot?

1. They ate real food. Processed foods filled with sugar and grains filled with phytic acid (which destroy tooth enamel) were not in their diet.

---

[20] https://www.byte.com/community/resources/article/oral-health-body-connection/

2. They took care of their teeth through natural means. Evidence has been found in Egyptian tombs dating back to 3000 B.C. that they chewed on sticks or rubbed them against their gums.
3. Many cultures practiced oil pulling (swishing a healthy oil around in your mouth).

Betty was a client who adopted this simple hygiene practice. She reported on a conversation with her dentist, who exclaimed: "What are you doing? Your gum health is amazing!" Betty proudly told her how I had introduced her to oil pulling, which she had been doing for several months. And Betty told me, "My gums have stopped bleeding when I brush and floss. My teeth aren't sensitive like they used to be. They are getting whiter! And food is tasting great!"

The *Journal of Ayurveda and Integrative Medicine* highlighted a study that reviewed holistic approaches to oral health and discovered that oil pulling is one of the most effective natural health solutions known to scientists, preventing tooth decay and loss, and curing more than 30 systemic diseases.[21]

> *"Health is like money. We never have a true idea of its value until we lose it."*
>
> —Josh Billings

The Healing Power of Oil Pulling

Oil pulling is simple and easy and quick. You just put one teaspoon of coconut oil in your mouth. Coconut oil has anti-bacterial, anti-fungal, and anti-viral properties that help eliminate the buildup of toxins. You can also use organic sesame oil, which has a calming effect if you deal with anxiety.

---

[21] References Dr Axe., e Whole Journey Self-care, integrative medicine

Coconut oil tastes good (don't swallow) and melts quickly. As it does, gently pull the oil through your teeth in a sucking and pushing action rather than swishing like you would with mouth wash. After about 5 minute of this (or more), rinse your mouth with water and spit several times. That's it!

Oil pulling removes bacteria and fungus. It helps make your teeth whiter, your gums healthier, and your breath fresher. Oil pulling also stimulates the immune system to fight toxins in the mouth and prevents them from finding their way into our bloodstream. This safe, simple practice is essential if you have ever had a root canal or are experiencing any type of mouth infection.

And, it only takes 5 minutes a day!

Food Choice of the Week

I will feature one recipe in each succeeding chapter, so you can begin to experiment with healthy cuisine as you read. This week it's a super delicious dessert:

APPLE CINNAMON CHIA PUDDING

INGREDIENTS
- 2 cups unsweetened coconut milk or almond milk
- 1/2 cup chia seeds
- Dash of vanilla
- 2-4 dashes of cinnamon
- Liquid stevia to taste (start with 10 drops and add more if needed)
- 1 apple, peeled and diced

PREPARATION

Combine all the ingredients (except the apple) in a glass jar or container and shake or stir with a whisk. Place in the refrigerator and shake or whisk again after 30 minutes and be sure to break up any clumps. After a couple of hours, the chia seeds will have soaked up most of the milk and your pudding will be ready to eat. Top with the chopped apple.

Eating apples demands a lot of chewing and when you spend time chewing you are sending signals to your brain telling your body that you have had enough to eat.

Apples reduce blood fats, and the fiber and phytonutrients help reduce the risk of heart disease, and lowers LDL cholesterol in the blood. But, best of all, apples improve gut health, which is the subject of our next chapter.

A study conducted at the New Zealand Institute for Plant and Food Research Limited demonstrated that the polyphenol-content of apples can help influence the bacterial population in the gut, resulting in reduced levels of inflammation and improved gastrointestinal health.

And, cinnamon? I love, love, love Cinnamon. What's not to love? Here's what cinnamon does in the body. It:

- Fights infection.
- Increases the metabolism.
- Stimulates healthy changes at a cellular level.
- Is high in fiber.
- Balances blood sugar helping with insulin resistance.

Remember to eat with your Caregiver mindset, count your chews, and experiment with Oil Pulling. See you in the next chapter where we head to the second vital region of the body, your gut.

Exercise

Although this chapter provides more detail on nutrition, I also mentioned movement, which is superpower number six. Your exercise for this week is to become more conscious of your movement patterns. Notice how much you sit every day. Begin to insert movement breaks throughout the day. Even a moment or two standing up and stretching can make a big difference.

What really makes a difference is to develop a daily routine, like stretching every morning before you do everything else. Remember, stagnation is sickness. Keep things moving and you'll help your body do the rest.

CHAPTER 10

YOUR BODY'S NATURAL DETOXIFICATION SYSTEM

> *"People are like stained - glass windows. They sparkle and shine when the sun is out, but when the darkness sets in, their true beauty is revealed only if there is a light from within."*
>
> —Elisabeth Kubler-Ross

In a prior chapter I introduced the Beautiful Healthy Body Blueprint and promised to get into the details later. Now's the time. I mentioned that the three most important physical factors determining a healthy, beautiful body are detoxification, gut health, and hormone balancing. So, in this chapter, we'll discuss detoxification.

How do we get healthy and stay healthy? One vitally important ingredient is learning how to deal with the toxic environment we live in. As I mentioned in chapter four, there's no escaping toxins! Each year, industries release about 10 million tons (21 billion pounds) of toxic chemicals into our environment. That works out to over 600 pounds every second. Two million tons are recognized carcinogens and almost 150 pounds of these become part of our environment every second.[22]

---

[22] https://www.worldometers.info/view/toxchem/

Some toxins we just can't escape, like breathing air polluted by car fumes and industrial waste blasted into the atmosphere and soil. Then there are all the antibiotics and pesticides in our food. Hopefully, we check labels but not everything is listed. And there are surprises. For instance, did you know that farm raised fish are toxic? The crowded conditions they are grown in make them sick, so antibiotics are used to offset disease and keep the fish alive until harvest time. Pesticides are also administered to keep away sea lice who show up in the unsanitary close quarters those fish swim in.

When it comes to the pesticides on our fruits and vegetables, did you know that those pesticides are waterproof? They are designed that way so that rainwater won't wash them off. But this also means that just rinsing them in the sink does nothing to remove the chemicals.

This means that it's very important to wash fruit and vegetables in water with vinegar to detox them.

Here's another not-so-fun fact: Did you know that there are an estimated 700 toxins inside your body right now? New-born babies arrive with almost 300 chemicals in the umbilical cord. Toxins harm our cells, causing inflammation, clogging up our livers, preventing our bodies from shedding unwanted belly fat and aging us prematurely. About 420 of these chemicals are known cancer causing agents.[23]

What's Not Working

Despite marvelous advances in medical science, we suffer from more chronic diseases today than ever before.

This, despite having more doctors and nurses, more healthcare practitioners, more gyms, more nutritionists, more dietitians, and more health education available than ever before in history.

---

[23] https://www.theworldcounts.com/challenges/toxic-exposures/polluted-bodies/chemicals-in-the-human-body

In my practice with clients, I'm seeing more serious diseases, even in younger people, then I have in all my 31 years of practice. I see auto immune diseases, neurological problems, dementia, Alzheimer's, mental health problems, and a vast array of unexplained aliments.

At the same time that we're at the forefront of a revolution in regenerative holistic medicine, the average life expectancy in the United States just had its biggest two-year decline in over 100 years. Experts now predict that the current generation of U.S. children are predicted to be the first to live shorter lives than their parents.[24]

Let that sink in!

How is this possible? Well, the quality of food that our depleted soil is grown in and the amount of chemicals and toxins we ingest must be at least part of the problem. These toxins arrive in food, water, air, and in the products we use on our skin and hair. This constant toxic exposure is causing serious harm to our cells and tissues and there is little we can do to insulate ourselves from them, short of living in a hazmat suit!

Wait, There's Some Good News

While we don't have much control over limiting the toxins in our environment, we *can* do something to get them out of our bodies. We do that through what's known as detoxification, of "detoxing." Simply put, detoxing supports the body's natural ways of eliminating toxins from the body. The detoxing process involves the liver, kidneys, lungs, colon, gut, lymphatic system, and skin.

> *"A detox is your opportunity to give your body a break and allow your own self-cleansing and self-healing processes to kick into gear"*
>
> —Food Matters

---

[24] https://www.health.harvard.edu/blog/why-life-expectancy-in-the-us-is-falling-202210202835

The liver is the largest fat burning organ and the primary organ responsible for filtration. It processes and filters the toxins from the blood and converts them into less harmful substances that can be eliminated from the body. When your liver processes these toxins, they get excreted through bile into the small intestine. But if those toxins are not bound to something, most will get reabsorbed in the gut through "enterohepatic recirculation." This explains why detoxification is needed to stay healthy, even when we eat a perfect diet.

The kidneys also play a vital role in detoxification by filtering waste and toxins from the blood and secreting them into urine. Our kidneys remove excess water and divert acid produced by the cells. Their job is to balance the fluid, salt, and mineral content in our bodies.

The lungs remove toxins in the form of carbon dioxide, sulfates nitrates, and other gases. They do this through respiration. That's breathing, something we do all the time. But many of us are shallow breathers, which limits the lungs detoxing process.

The lymphatic system includes the lymph nodes and their vessels. These help to remove toxins from our body's tissues and organs. This system also filters and traps viruses, bacteria, and toxins that could cause infection.

The skin is our largest detox organ and it removes toxins through sweating and fevers. When we wear synthetic clothing, we inhibit this process. Our skin can easily get clogged; chemical cosmetics are also harmful.

The colon absorbs nutrients and excretes waste. Our gut is the first line of defense against everything we put in our bodies. When our gut cannot handle the toxic overload that results from a poor diet and insufficient exercise (stagnation), liver absorption is severely impaired, and the other detox organs do not get enough nutrients to work properly.

What Can We Do to Help?

Knowing what's in our food and choosing only toxin free products keeps some toxins and heavy metals out of our bodies. But this doesn't address the environmental toxics we can't avoid. So, knowing that we are, inevitably, dealing with toxins, we can begin to watch for signs of brewing problems and take early action.

Some of the signs our body gives us that it needs a detox:
- Low energy. Dragging yourself through the day, especially in the afternoon.
- Excess weight. You just can't lose those extra pounds.
- Overeating. Never feeling "full" or satisfied.
- Insomnia. Struggling to fall asleep and waking up throughout the night.
- Skin conditions. Rashes, psoriasis, eczema, dandruff, etc.
- Brain fog. Struggling to focus and forgetting.
- Constipation and/or loose stools.
- Bloating and being gassy.
- Diminished sex drive.
- Sugar cravings throughout the day.
- Persistent headaches.
- Daily mood swings.

You need a break on the weekends, right? So does your body. It needs time to recharge, just like you do. A body that doesn't get enough rest becomes run down over time from the increasing load of toxins that aren't eliminated. This includes whatever not-so-healthy foods we eat regularly, the caffeine and alcohol, lack of exercise, unhealthy mental states (like self-judgment and chronic anxiety), plus the insidious impact of stress.

A properly executed "detox" gives our kidneys, liver, skin, colon, and lungs a reduced workload, rest time, and the right conditions to deal with everything that runs our systems down, restoring much-needed balance and vitality to our body.

Detoxing your body is actually quite easy. In fact, you're not even doing it, your body is. What *we* do is support the body to do its thing. Here's how we can help the body detox itself:

1. Drink spring water (drink half your weight in ounces of water every day).
2. Start your day with 16 ounces of room temperature water with half the juice of a lemon.
3. Green tea is healthy. It does have caffeine so drink early in the day.
4. Avoid processed food. That includes everything in a box, bag, or can, and anything that has a shelf life.
5. Eat two cups of green vegetables a day, raw, steamed, or sautéed. Herbs are great for detoxing, (cilantro, parsley, basil, and mint are some of my favorites)
6. Avoid products with chemicals and synthetic ingredients.
7. Take good quality supplements like omega 3 and magnesium. If you need a dependable source these are my favorite visit resource: https://soniamarie.beyuna.com
8. Manage stress by taking a 15 minute break every day to decompress.
9. Maintain a regular bedtime and ensure you have 7-8 hours of sleep per night.
10. Exercise and sweat regularly. Far infrared saunas are wonderful for a detox.
11. Wash all your produce with plain white vinegar water and 1 tablespoon of baking soda, the best natural produce wash.
12. Read the labels and buy accordingly.

Fasting

We all fast every day or, rather, every night. We start eating again in the morning and we call that "break-fast." Our bodies rest and detox while we sleep. We can assist this process by learning the best timing for eating and fasting.

Intermittent fasting is the practice of limiting our feeding time to a set period of time every day. For instance, you might eat breakfast at 9am and finish dinner by 7. That adds up to an eating window of 10 hours, which means that you are effectively fasting – letting your body rest – for the other 14 hours.

Most of us have experienced what happens when we eat a big meal late at night. We don't sleep well and we wake up groggy. Our bodies struggled to digest and rest at the same time which is a formula for metabolic disaster. When we commit to a set eating window, we can avoid the binging that happens through unconscious choices (that pizza might look pretty good around midnight but …).

Benefits of Fasting

1. Promotes blood sugar control by reducing insulin resistance.
2. Promotes better health by fighting inflammation.
3. May enhance heart health by improving blood pressure, triglycerides, and cholesterol levels.
4. May boost brain function and prevent neurodegenerative disorders.
5. Aids weight loss by limiting calorie intake and boosting metabolism.
6. Increases growth hormone secretion, which is vital for growth, metabolism, weight loss, and muscle strength.
7. Could extend longevity.
8. May aid in cancer prevention and increase the effectiveness of chemotherapy.

Mary's Story

After a lifetime of depriving myself of food, then binging, then beating myself up over and over and repeating the same cycle, I was ready for a change. When I heard Sonia talking about food freedom and using food as medicine and how important detoxing was, I immediately knew she could help me. Over our three months working together, Sonia helped me understand how dangerous toxins are, how they were harming my day-to-day life, and how to get rid of them.

Sonia helped me change my relationship with food and my eating habits. Each week she added on a little more information so my program was always very doable. I learned which foods healed my gut and alkalized my body. I began to feel better immediately (I hadn't even realized how badly I was feeling!). My lower back pain completely subsided, and I began to sleep much better. I am forever grateful for all the wisdom Sonia has shared with me.

Detoxification is a vast subject, far beyond what we can cover in this book. Specific programs are detailed on my web site and explained in client sessions. You don't have to become a detox expert, just learn the basics to help your body help you have the happy, healthy life you deserve.

This chapter introduces a number of healthy practices – and that's superpower number seven, the last one and, in many ways, the most important one for long lasting improvement. We'll be covering more healthy practices in the remaining chapters, but I'd like you to consider beginning to think differently about everything you do. Is what you are doing a healthy practice or not? For instance, slumping on the coach binging Netflix is probably not a healthy practice. Stretching every morning before coffee is. And what about that coffee? Unless it's organic,or fairtrade clean sources, most of our coffee in America has got mold on it. And how much caffeine do you really need.

A new guiding question becomes:

Is what I am about to do or eat healthy or not?

Then we answer by activating superpower number four, choice, and what happens changes our future.

CHAPTER 11

HEALING OUR GUT

"What kills us isn't one big thing, but thousands of tiny obligations we can't turn down for fear of disappointing others."

—Alain de Botton

Tina came to me asking if I could help her reduce the pain in her hands and feet, lower cholesterol, lower her blood pressure, help with her sleep, lose weight, and balance her hormones. A tall order, right? No, not really! Most people think that their symptoms are disconnected and need to be taken care of one by one. This seems overwhelming, especially when we have lots of responsibilities, managing work, households, finances, and family. But there's one common thread, a single health issue at the heart of most disease symptoms: an unhealthy gut.

Before we consider foods and practices for healing the gut, let's study Tina's primary nutritional situation, which as you'll remember is always emotionally based. In this case, Tina showed up with a big obligation problem. This presented in two primary ways.

The Friend Problem

Tina was a very hard worker and always had been. She had earned multiple degrees and sat at the top of her nursing profession. She worked odd hours, long shifts in very stressful situations.

Tina loved going out with her girlfriends and they went to Disney Land twice every month. She had a season pass and they had been going for years. Her days off were for play, unrestricted, uncommitted, doing whatever she wanted, a reward for all her hard work. So, she ate crappy food and enjoyed Happy Hour. Over time, this contributed to that long list of health problems.

Although Tina felt she was "being bad" when she was with her friends, it was a well-earned escape and she felt that she had no other choice. How could she give up all of her favorite Disneyland foods and happy hours with her friends when they depended on her to share those fun experiences? She told me, "This is the one thing I looked forward to and LOVE TO DO: eat all that fried food, lots of coffee flavored drinks and desserts and treats!" But this is what was giving her the pain, anxiety, insomnia, brain fog, etc. Yes, it was the junk food, but it was her feeling of obligation that drove her to eat that way.

The Family Problem

Tina was a rule follower. As the eldest child, it had been her responsibility to set a perfect example. It was also a feature of her culture to study and extend her education. So, not only was she working full time for very long hours with little sleep, she was also studying for a Master's degree. When I asked her if she was excited to be nearing completion, she exclaimed, "No! I didn't even want to do this Master's program." She went on to confess that this was just another family obligation.

Every time she saw her parents, her mom would harass her about her excess weight, which made her feel guilty and ashamed. But her mom would also force feed her snacks and desserts and, if she resisted, would complain that she was dishonoring her mother and their culture. Tina felt trapped in obligation and that she couldn't win.

Expectations imposed on us and the obligations
we feel to friends and family can drive unhealthy choices.

The Gut Healing Method

I introduced Tina to the concept of gut health. As I told her (and every other client) our gut holds the key to health and determines how our body feels. In fact, it is no exaggeration to say that healing your gut is a virtual passport to more youthful energy, an ideal body shape, proper hormone and brain function, optimal digestion, and a strong immune system. An unhealthy gut microbiome causes unwanted weight gain, high blood sugar, high cholesterol and multiple chronic diseases like obesity, diabetes, migraine headaches, IBS, SIBO, PCOS, heart disease, cancers, Alzheimer, dementia, etc.

Your gut houses over 80% of your immune system. It also controls many important aspects of health, like proper brain function, mood, sleep cycles, digestion, energy, and metabolism. Serotonin, dopamine, and melatonin are manufactured in your gut. These are your "happy" motivational support hormones, your blood pressure regulators, and your sleep cycle internal clock hormones.

Good gut health has been proven over and over again to regulate
our mood, skin issues, manage brain fog, anxiety and depression.

But there is considerable misinformation out there on how to heal the gut. Many supposedly "gut healthy" foods, including fermented vegetables, actually harm your gut health, if they are heavily processed, and stored in tin cans or plastics with toxic preservatives added.

Fermented / Probiotic and Prebiotic Foods – The Good Ones

The good news is that properly fermented foods can be your golden ticket to gut health. They can also be incredibly tasty. Our gut is home to trillions of bacteria cells, some of them good and some of them bad. These are called probiotics. Healthy, fermented foods can quickly restore balance in the gut by supporting the growth of the good ones and eliminating the bad ones.

Here's more good news. What are called "prebiotics" feed probiotics and help protect our gastrointestinal system, central nervous system, immune system, and cardiovascular system. Increasing the number of prebiotic-containing foods in the diet may help with:

- Regulating blood sugar levels
- Maintaining a healthy weight
- Reducing blood lipids
- Supporting healthy intestinal motility
- Feeding beneficial gut bacteria

I taught Tina how to make her own fermented foods and she was amazed how easy it actually was.

Then, simply adding in one or two servings every day literally changed her life. She was thrilled to discover that she didn't need to lose her social life or quit enjoying eating. These new foods tasted delicious, so good that she actually *wanted* to eat them – which was the opposite of dutifully eating what she thought she should.

> *Her gut started to heal. She began to feel better and her skin looked amazing.*

This is what happens when you follow The Gut Healing Method. Why? Because the toxins in your body are quickly cleansed, as the bad bacteria in your gut die off. Like Tina, you will begin to feel positive changes in your body and your energy will increase as the good bacteria become dominant again.

You are what you eat, and you are also what you eat eats!

Here is the basic, easy process for making your own fermented foods, including pickled carrots, cucumbers (dill, sweet, pickles), and sauerkraut.

What you will need

- Salt. Kosher, sea salt, Celtic salt, or Himalayan salt will do, just be sure it's not plain table salt and that it's not been iodized.
- **Starter Liquid** - ¼ cup of liquid from a previous batch (for the first time you can use organic sauerkraut from the store.
- **Filtered water.**

FERMENTING VEGETABLES

- Slice veggies thin ½ slices.
- Add 1/4 cup of a starter culture (the juice from a previous ferment such as homemade sauerkraut. If you don't have a starter culture, add 1 tablespoon salt.
- Using the bottom of a wooden spatula, push down the veggies to eliminate air pockets. The goal is a tightly packed jar.
- Once your jar is full, add the remaining liquid from the bowl so your veggies are covered with liquid.
- Add a lid, NOT airtight, and leave the jar out on the counter for three days.

After 5-10 days, taste the veggies to see if the flavors have developed. Once you're happy with the flavor, transfer to your refrigerator.

Here are a few recipes to experiment with, just to get you started.

LEMON/LIME GINGER CARROTS

(add to salads, sandwiches, soups, or as a side)

(Fermented Carrots are helpful for anxiety, adrenal fatigue, and tummy sensitivities.)

- **Carrots** 3 large
- **Fresh ginger** (2 inches of ginger)
- **Zest and juice of 1 whole Lemon & Lime**
- **Above Basic Fermentation Recipe**

PICKLES

- **Cucumbers 4 Medium**
- Peppercorns 1 TBSP
- Bay leaves 2 whole leaves
- Garlic-2 whole cloves
- Dill 2 TBSP Fresh
- **Above Basic Fermentation Recipe**

SAUERKRAUT

- **Fennel Seed 1 TBSP**
- **Cumin Seed 1 TBSP**
- **Coriander Seed 1TBSP**
- **Above Basic Fermentation Recipe**

FRUIT PREBIOTICS

(for toppings, yogurt, desserts or sides)

QUICK CRANBERRY APPLE SAUCE

- 2 apples, chopped (organic)
- 2 oranges, chopped
- 2 cups cranberries, fresh or frozen chopped.
- 1 cup pineapple chopped
- 1/2 cup pecans, chopped (or nut of choice)
- 1/2 cup apple cider (or apple juice, plus more if needed)
- 1/4 cup maple syrup (or honey, monk fruit sugar or stevia)
- 1/2 cup kombucha, or kefir (this is your starter liquid)
- 1 tsp salt

The Method

- Chop apples, cranberries, oranges, pineapple and nuts and add to a large bowl.
- Stir in the apple cider, and maple syrup or sweetener of choice.
- Pour kefir or starter liquid over the chopped mixture and sprinkle with salt. Then stir to combine and add to a quart-sized mason jar or glass bottle.
- Pack your mixture down into the jar and top with apple cider until all food pieces are covered.
- Cover with an airtight mason jar lid and set at room temperature. 2-4 times a day, burp your jar and give it a turn or two.
- After 2 days, transfer to the refrigerator. Enjoy!

CHERRY VANILLA KOMBUCHA

- 1 quart unflavored kombucha
- 1 cups of Fresh or frozen Cherries, Organic is preferred (you can also use strawberries or watermelon)
- 1 tsp vanilla extract

The Method
- Place cherries (or fruit of choice, after cleaning it well) in the bottom of a clean quart jar.
- Pour in vanilla extract.
- Pour in kombucha until the jar is full.
- Cap the jar tight with a two-part jar lid.
- Leave on a countertop in a warm room. Periodically check the pop-top on the lid. If it no longer pops, burp the jar by releasing a bit of air out of it, and then screw the cap back on tight.
- After 4-5 days on the counter, your kombucha should be showing bubbles and signs of carbonation. At this point, you can transfer your kombucha into a bottle, or leave it in the jar then refrigerate, Enjoy with in 2 weeks.

SODA

Use 2 TBSP in a 6-ounce glass of seltzer water for a healthy Soda.

As Tina found (and you will too) these delicious dishes pack a powerful punch. Adding them to your diet is an easy way to enjoy gut healing foods that are delicious. You and your family can enjoy them in yogurts, cereals, bread, biscuits, and drinks.

"I didn't realize how bad I was feeling until I started to feel good," is something I often hear often from my clients. This makes my heart sing!

Exercise

The Food Exchange

Here's your exercise for the week.

1. Pick one food that you really enjoy but have been told you shouldn't eat and decide that, temporarily, you won't eat it until you decide it's safe to bring it back into your diet.

2. Now, substitute something that is close to what you want but is a healthier option (I have thousands of amazing tasting healthy recipes, all available here www.soniamarienutrition.com).
3. Tell yourself: "I'm an adult. I can eat the food I want. I'm choosing a healthier option and feel that I can have my desired food after, when I'm feeling better or have hit my goal. It's not that I shouldn't eat it, but it's just not aligned with what I really want right now. My choice is that I want to try this other option. This is my choice!"

And as you begin on this journey, choosing what you want that empowers you and making your own healthy food, remember these three life saving tips:

1. Food is your medicine.
2. Every healthy step takes you further down the healing road.
3. Small changes yield big results quickly.

CHAPTER 12

BALANCING OUR HORMONES

*Hormones get no respect. We think of them as
the elusive chemicals that make us a bit moody, but
these magical little molecules do so much more.*

—Susannah Cahalan

What do we know about our hormones? Most of us know the basics, for instance, that if our metabolism isn't working properly then we can't lose weight. But, other than that, hormones seem to be a great mystery.

We start figuring it out when we turn 50 and our body stops working properly, especially when our curves change. My clients call it "square shape," or they tell me, "I look like a sausage," when I ask them about their body type. We laugh, but it's not really that funny because quite beyond how we look is how we feel and the chronic diseases that may be brewing under the surface.

Hormones 101

Hormones coordinate vital functions in our body. They carry messages through the blood to organs, skin, muscles, and other tissues, signaling the body to do what it needs to do, when it needs to do it. Did you know there are over 50 hormones in the body? Here's a short list of what they control:

- Metabolism.
- Homeostasis (constant internal balance).
- Growth and development.
- Sexual function.
- Reproduction.
- Sleep-wake cycle.
- Mood regulation.

Hormone balance is crucial for heart health, for thyroid balance... for so many functions. A hormonal imbalance is basically too much or too little. Even slightly too much or too little of a hormone can cause major changes to your body that might require treatment.

Some hormonal imbalances are temporary while others are chronic. Some may require treatment while others may not significantly impact your health but *may* negatively affect your quality of life.

Food enters our stomach to be digested and absorbed into our blood stream. The blood is what creates our cells, our tissues, our organs, even contributes to our thoughts. For instance, we think differently when we eat meat than when we eat broccoli. We feel differently when we drink coffee or alcohol than when we consume sugar. Eating affects our hormones and hormones affect our moods, motivating us or discouraging us.

If you are feeling any of these symptoms, then you should investigate balancing your hormones.

- Brain fog, migraines, headaches, insomnia.
- Ovarian cysts, fibroids, acne, cellulite, or other skin conditions.
- Bloating, bowel issues, weight fluctuations.

- Endocrine disruptors like cycle irregularities, painful menstruation, early or late menopause, fertility issues.

History of infections, chronic immune challenges, or have been diagnosed with conditions such as endometriosis or polycystic ovary syndrome (PCOS).

How does it work?

Some of my clients do a Hormone Balancing program with me and we break it down into four phases over four weeks. 1) Reducing inflammation Phase 2) Detoxifying Phase 3) Absorption & Reeducating Phase 4) Healing Phase. You can find more details on my website at www.soniamarienutrition.com

Here are three tips for cleansing and balancing our hormones:

Tip# 1 - Balancing Stress levels

Adaptogens are really helpful. For instance, ashwagandha or reishi can help with stress reduction, as can activities like meditation or journaling in the morning. These calming activities help your body deal with cortisol levels in a healthy way and help your body produce female hormones like estrogen and progesterone.

Tip # 2 - Liver Support & Proper Bile Flow

Fiber is vitally important for hormonal balance. Mom was right; we should eat our veggies! Cruciferous vegetables, like broccoli and cauliflower, bok choy, and kale contain phytonutrients that help break down and detox excess estrogen. Men are now developing higher levels of estrogen in their bodies because of poor quality foods, like deli meats, added sugar, eggs, etc.

Tip #3 - Eating Healthy Fat

Eating the right kinds of fats make a big difference in hormone health and help you regulate your sexy hormones like estrogen and progesterone. You can add more hormone-friendly fats to your diet like:

- fatty fish
- eggs
- avocado
- coconut
- olive oil
- nuts and seeds

Healthy fats also help to balance blood sugar and promote insulin sensitivity, which is especially important for women with Polycystic ovary syndrome (PCOS), and for successfully losing weight.

"I just can't seem to make myself do it!"

Liz showed up in my office and said, "I wish I had more motivation or willpower or maybe I'm just weak or lazy!" She called it emotional eating, stress eating, and bored eating.

Any kind of eating that creates worry, stress, shame and blame will create a constant struggle and decrease self-compassion. Liz assured me that she didn't think she could give up her morning coffee and the sandwich she has for lunch each day, and she definitely couldn't give up her sweets after dinner and, by the way, giving up the occasional glass of wine at the end of the week after a long work week? Not going to happen.

This was her reward. I just smiled at Liz and said" I got cha! I know that you feel like this is going to be such a challenge, and it seems difficult to even want to start. But, we do not need to take everything away all at once." I showed Liz how to start small and take small steps to build a healthy daily routine.

Building that healthy daily routine is essential for creating the life that you want. Actually, it *all* comes down to your daily habits. Because we are all busy and multitasking to the 10th degree. We must stay focused on a plan.

Small steps can bring big success.

There's a saying: "If you fail to plan, you are planning to fail!" To stay healthy, we must plan, we must set some non-negotiable rules for ourselves. These non-negotiables have kept me and my clients strong and healthy for years.

Let's Start Young

I truly believe that helping our children understand food and getting them into the kitchen early is crucial for their health and wellbeing. Introducing new foods in creative ways is necessary for their gut health and metabolism.

Eat the rainbow, I'm sure you've heard this before. What does it mean, and why is it important? The color of food—its pigmentation—indicates the specific nutrients that produce can offer you, health-wise.

We all want to cook healthy food for our family. But, how? How do you get a picky eater to eat vegetables. This is usually a question I get from moms. I decided to help one of my mom clients learn how to feed her kids healthy food because she really wanted to make a positive difference in her daughter and her son's health.

Her daughter had ADHD and her son had a lot of food sensitivities. So, I decided to put together a kids cooking class! We had 11 kids ages 5-13 come to that class. Actually, I did what I call a reverse cooking class.

First, I welcomed the kids and handed out colorful aprons and lemonade, then I fed them treats, so they thought… I gave them yogurt, and then mac-n-cheese, then chicken tenders, and for dessert we had brownies with chocolate frosting.

I walked around asking if they would like to learn how to cook the foods they ate. I received an overall "Can we have seconds first? then a "YESSSSSSSS, we want to cook this kind of food."

> *The mom's sat in awe as they watched their little ones literally lick their plates.*

As we gathered around the island to start cooking, the kids started telling "I don't like that vegetable, or that one. I don't like oats, then, I don't like avocado," and so on and so on. I suggested that we should not decide we don't like something until we try it.

And, that everything they said they didn't like they had just gobbled up! They were shocked and became excited to find out how I did it. So, I exposed the healthy ingredients (after they enjoyed eating, concept-free!).

We had enjoyed carrot yogurt, butternut squash mac-n-cheese, (dairy free), chicken tenders battered with oats and spices that were baked and crispy, and brownies with frosting made from avocado and sweet potato. They were thrilled and all the kids took doggie bags home to share with their family.

It's all about starting with foods that have the right flavor and texture, in familiar recipes they already enjoy. I call that "The Naughty Nice Way," eating foods that we believe are naughty that taste great and are actually healthy!

Action Step

This will start you on a path of food prepping and commitment to building support for your healthy lifestyle with others. It is important to build a support system with family and friends.

Invite a friend to lunch or dinner and take great care preparing the meal for them. Keep it simple and make something easy. Like this amazing recipe below. Nourish your bodies (*and freak out your taste buds*) with this yummy salmon dish! Supercharged with ingredients that are rich in healthy fats, nutrients, and anti-inflammatory compounds, it's the perfect meal to support your hormone levels and lift your energy. Not to mention, it is wickedly delicious!

SALMON FLORENTINE

Ingredients

2 servings
- 2 teaspoons Extra Virgin Olive Oil
- 2 Garlic (cloves, sliced)
- 1/4 cup Shallot (chopped)
- 8 Cremini Mushrooms (sliced)
- 1 TBSP Capers
- ½ Lemon (juiced)
- 1 3/4 cups Canned Coconut Milk
- 2 tsps Thyme (fresh)
- Sea Salt & Black Pepper (to taste)
- 12 ozs Salmon Fillet (skinless)
- 2 cups Baby Spinach

Directions
1. Add the oil, garlic, and shallots to a large skillet and sauté until fragrant, about two to three minutes.
2. Then, add the mushrooms and continue sautéing until the mushrooms are browned, about five to seven minutes. Add the lemon juice to the pan to deglaze.
3. Add the coconut milk, thyme, salt, and pepper. Stir well and bring the sauce to a gentle simmer. Add the salmon pieces,

nestling them into the sauce. Cover and cook for five minutes or until the salmon is cooked to your desired doneness.
4. Add the spinach to the sauce for a few minutes until wilted. Divide evenly between bowls and enjoy!
5. Optional: Can be served over quinoa, gluten free noodles, or rice.

Here are some of the key ingredients and why they might give you a new way to look at your food and ingredients:

Salmon: Wild caught salmon is an excellent source of omega-3 fatty acids. Omega-3s support a healthy metabolism, reduce inflammation, and balance hormone levels. These fatty acids are also essential for maintaining good brain health.

Capers: Capers are rich in quercetin, a flavonoid that has anti-inflammatory properties. Consuming quercetin has been shown to reduce the risk of developing reproductive cancers, meaning capers can assist in maintaining hormone health.

Avocado Oil: is rich in monounsaturated fatty acids and has both anti-inflammatory and antioxidant qualities. It has a glycemic index of zero and contains zero carbohydrates, making it a diabetic-friendly oil.

Avocado oil helps lower LDL cholesterol and increase HDL cholesterol. As a result, it helps to improve heart health and decreases the risk of coronary diseases. In addition, avocado oil has anti- inflammatory properties, which help prevent damage in the walls of arteries caused by plaque buildup.

Fiber

It is important to choose higher fiber foods. Adequate dietary fiber intake is associated with several health benefits including better digestive health and Reducing inflammation. This meal is grain-free, gluten-free, and uses low glycemic ingredients.

A 2018 research review found that prebiotic fiber, like that in garlic and onions, may be even better for your gut than the fiber in some fruits, vegetables and whole grains.

Antioxidants

Vitamin A & Vitamin C support various cellular functions of our immune system, reduce oxidative stress in cells, and are useful in the treatment of inflammatory diseases. This recipe is packed with vitamin A such as Thyme, spinach. Vitamin C from Lemon.

Iron

Iron is an important mineral that helps produce red blood cells and transports oxygen throughout the body and is a common nutrient-deficiency in plant-based diets. This dish incorporates iron-rich foods like greens like spinach, and iron sources are paired with citrus foods that have vitamin C to enhance iron absorption.

B Vitamins

These vitamins help enzymes release energy from carbohydrates and fat, break down amino acids, and transport oxygen and energy-containing nutrients around the body. This meal (above) provides B vitamins from green leafy vegetables.

Resource:https://academic.oup.com/ibdjournal/article/20/4/732/4579035 & Cambridge.org, FOODMATTERS.COM

CHAPTER 13

COMMITMENT TO HEALTH

"There is a difference between interest and commitment. When you're interested in doing something, you do it only when circumstances permit. When you're committed to something, you accept no excuses, only results."

—Art Turock

Here's why I love health coaching and what I've identified as the single greatest contributor to achieving break through and lasting results: Commitment.

Most people understand that we need to be healthy to have a happy life. But making a *commitment* to become truly healthy and then doing what's necessary to follow through to get those results… that's what I get to see my clients doing every day. Of course, I also hear every reason under the sun why "I can't." That conversation starts like this: "It's my lifestyle. I just can't handle it all. Every day revolves around family, work, and entertaining. There's just no time left for all this health stuff."

This is exactly the opposite of commitment, what I call "self-sabotage." It's a common and primary reason why having a health coach can make the difference between vibrant health into the senior years and lingering chronic illness even at an early age.

Making the commitment to become healthy changes everything.

Choosing health activates Superpower # 4.

Adopting a holistic approach brings advantages you just have to experience to understand. But making big changes on your own can be difficult, often because you don't know where to start. This is why having someone to guide your journey is invaluable. Let's eavesdrop on a consultation with one of my clients:

Debbie: "Well, I've been struggling with my weight for years. I've tried so many diets and I do lose some weight but then I gain it all back, plus some. I feel like I'm constantly yo-yoing with my weight."

Me: "That's very common. Can you tell me about your eating habits?"

Debbie: "I eat a lot of junk food, especially when I'm stressed out or feeling down. I know it's not good for me, but I just can't stop. I also have a hard time eating enough vegetables and other healthy foods."

Me: "Okay, and how's your energy level?"

Debbie: "It's really low. I feel tired all the time, even when I get enough sleep. I also have trouble falling asleep and staying asleep."

Me: "I see. Well, it sounds like there are underlying issues to address. Let's start with increasing how much water you drink every day, OK? We'll add more whole foods and reduce processed foods. I'll also give you two or three strategies for dealing with stress that don't involve food. How does that sound?"

Debbie: "Really? That sounds so … manageable. And I really do need to make changes. You know, I think I can do this!"

Me: "Yes, you can. We'll start small and build new behaviors. We'll work in phases, with measurable goals for each week. We'll also look at your sleep habits. Poor sleep can affect your weight and energy levels. Finally, we'll work on creating new, healthy habits you can maintain over the long term. That yo-yo dieting can be really hard on your body and your mental health too. So, we want to help you make changes that you can stick with for life."

Debbie: "OK. That sounds like a plan. I'm ready."

How Health Coaches Help

We know that having a trainer helps us in the gym. Working with a health coach is even more beneficial. They can keep us accountable for achieving our wellness goals and making steady progress. By having someone there to support, motivate, and keep us on the right path, it's easier to stay committed, even during the tough times. Like, when the scale doesn't seem to change fast enough, which can happen.

Of course, you need a coach that you really resonate with, someone who has the expertise and knowledge to help you navigate the complexities of holistic nutrition and lifestyle practices but also someone you connect with personally. And there's no one-size-fits all program.

True health coaching is always customized for each individual, supporting them to make informed decisions to improve the health of their uniquely personal body, mind, and spirit.

It has to be that personal in my practice because we identify the root causes of a person's particular aliments to discover the unique needs and obstacles to addressing them effectively. And that takes trust. Since no two people are remotely the same, I craft a plan tailored specifically for each person, helping them meet their goals quickly and efficiently and - surprisingly to my clients – in ways that turn out to be enjoyable!

Here are comments from three clients who reversed major diseases and healed with food medicine.

"Working with Sonia Marie was an absolute game-changer for my health and wellness journey. Her holistic approach to nutrition not only helped me transform my body, she also helped me finally balance my cholesterol levels that were high for 28 years. I was actually able to get off my medication! Sonia Marie's program transformed my entire life and my family's lives. Her personalized guidance and support helped me to make sustainable changes to my diet and lifestyle that have had a profound impact on my overall well-being. I can't recommend her strongly enough!"

—Debbie L.

"Sonia Marie is an absolute gem in the world of nutrition / wellbeing. Her holistic approach not only helped me achieve my weight-loss goals but also completely transformed my relationship with my body and with food. I've had a lifetime of issues with emotional eating but, incredibly, that's over! Her step-by-step system has been invaluable to my health journey, and I will always be grateful for her impact on my life."

—Roxanne C.

"I'm beyond grateful for my experience working with Sonia Marie. Her expertise in holistic nutrition helped me get back to living my life again. When I showed up at her office, I was in so much pain! And everything I ate made me feel miserable. I had stopped going out with friends because I was so embarrassed! I didn't know what was causing it and I'd been struggling for three years. No one could give me any answers.

"Sonia Marie knew exactly what was going on. She developed a personalized eating and healing plan for me that felt manageable and enjoyable. With her guidance, I learned how to nourish my

body by supporting my gut health. I've never felt better, both physically and mentally! Thank you, for giving me my life back!"

—Lynn J.

While their situations were different and what I offered them varied, I helped all of them activate their fourth superpower, the power of choice. As you'll soon learn, I really feel that this is most important superpower. Once it is online, you become the master of your destiny because every choice contributes to health or disease, happiness or discouragement.

Food *is* Medicine... and it can be Delicious!

NEWSFLASH: You don't have to give up taste in order to get healthy!

Once you start adding more whole foods into your diet, your taste buds revive. They become more sensitive to how delicious real, fresh ingredients taste. This means saying goodbye to bland salads and hello to delicious, nutritious meals!

Food is the fuel our bodies run on. We wouldn't put crappy fuel in our car, right? The same goes for the food we put in our body. It should never be cheap or of an inferior quality if we want our bodies to function optimally.

Consuming processed, chemical-laden, and nutrient-poor foods has immediate and long-lasting detrimental effects on our bodies. It causes inflammation, slows our digestion, lowers energy, and contributes to chronic illnesses. When we replace a poor diet with whole, nutrient dense foods, our bodies rebound fast. We are supporting them to fend off disease and lower inflammation.

Making the commitment to put quality first could add years to your life. More important, those years can be your best years, health-wise.

Healthy food has gotten a bad rap. Many people believe that if it's healthy it won't taste good, while "cheat foods" - the tasty ones that are bad for us, those guilty pleasures – always taste better.

Enough with the crazy!!!!!! Healthy food tastes great… when our taste buds come back to life. So, instead of thinking of good and bad foods, the ones we *should* eat vs the ones we *want* to eat, let's think about nutrition and garbage. Junk food is garbage! It's in the name! It's junk, it's garbage. Once we make our commitment to health and start changing or eating habits, we very quickly lose our interest in that crap. Real food is medicine, but *this* medicine is delicious!

Holistic Wellness – It Includes Your Brain

Holistic healthcare addresses all of you - mind, body, and spirit, to help you reach your maximum potential. Prioritizing brain health is a vital aspect of your commitment. Having a healthy mind improves physical wellbeing, just as regular exercise improves our emotional life and increases our energy levels.

When you consume healthy food, your brain works better. It receives the essential nutrients it requires to function optimally, improving mood, reducing stress, and turbo charging cognitive performance.

Here A Few Repercussions of Having A Healthy Brain

Energy

A healthy brain helps your body have the energy it needs for peak performance, helping you feel energized throughout the day and improving productivity and wellbeing.

Reduced Risk of Chronic Diseases

Clear thinking can lower the risk of developing chronic diseases like heart disease, diabetes, and cancer. How? You make better choices. Adopting healthy practices into your lifestyle means that you decrease inflammation in your body while strengthening immunity to infections and aiding natural detoxification and healing processes.

Improved Your Digestive Health

The way you think influences what you put on your plate and in your mouth. Digestion plays a vital role in improving everything. A diet rich in fiber, probiotics, and digestive enzymes enables your body to absorb nutrients more easily, reduce bloating, eliminate food sensitivities and allergies, and get rid of energy bandits! Choosing healthy food starts in a healthy brain.

Choosing Health

Here's how I guide my clients to choose and incorporate holistic practices into their everyday life, in seven easy steps:

1. Focus on eating whole and nutrient-dense foods, such as fresh fruits and vegetables, lean proteins sources, healthy fats, and whole grains.
2. Limit the consumption of processed and refined foods such as white bread, sugary drinks, and packaged snacks.
3. Hydration is essential; drink enough water each day to support optimal digestion and overall wellbeing (half your body weight in ounces).
4. Stay physically active by walking regularly, practicing yoga, and working out.
5. Develop mental wellness through mindfulness meditation therapy and regular time in nature.
6. Support local farmers whenever possible by purchasing organic, sustainable foods.
7. Engage with your community. This may involve volunteering, attending events, or just reaching out to friends and family for support.

Adopting food as medicine, embracing holistic nutrition, and committing to daily wellness practices are great for you personally and also create a profoundly positive effect on those around you and for our planet. As you become healthier and happier, you'll begin to inspire others into this simple but profound realization:

> *Who wouldn't want to feel their best and*
> *make a positive impact on society?*

I'm a Nutrition Nerd and Proud of It!

Given all the health challenges I've been through, I love finally feeling good! And I love showing my clients how powerful our bodies and minds are. Holistic nutrition and lifestyle practices offer us much more than improved health. It's about freedom! All the things we want to enjoy in life? Suddenly, we are free to really live!

When we say, "I choose to be healthy!" we're not just talking about deciding to losing weight. We are making a commitment to feel amazing, with no pain and plenty of energy. That's the goal and it's within reach. All it takes is commitment and follow through, with the support we need to give ourselves, our families, and the planet, the greatest gift of all: one more healthy, happy person contributing their best to society.

CHAPTER 14

RELATIONSHIPS THAT NURTURE OUR WELLBEING

*"A great relationship is about two things.
First, appreciating the similarities.
And second, respecting the differences."*

—Invajy

Relationships represent our third superpower. Healthy relationships provide emotional support, companionship, and a contribute to a sense of shared purpose and meaning in life while at the same time helping reduce stress, build social skills, and relieve depression.

We are always in relationship with someone, even if it's just ourselves, and the quality of those relationships affects our health in powerful ways. Sadly, we receive no education about this, but it's not difficult to quickly pick up what we need to know and do to develop healthy relationships that nurture us.

I always talk with my clients about the quality of their relationships.

Relationships play a fundamental role in shaping and sustaining our emotional and mental and even our physical well-being. Positive, healthy relationships also support our ongoing growth while negative, toxic, or abusive ones can damage us at every level and make us feel stuck in joyless states of anxiety and fear.

There are so many different kinds of relationships, but here are the major ones that can provide health supporting "nutrition" in our daily lives.

Family Relationships

These include our blood family - parents, siblings, grandparents, aunts/uncles/cousins – plus the extended family we gain through marriages. Positive family relations help develop our sense of identity, self-esteem, and worthiness within a small, personal, very defined "community." Feeling loved, valued, and appreciated within our family is a key determiner for mental and emotional wellbeing. Studies have also indicated that children growing up in loving, supportive families gain better cognitive, social, and emotional growth compared to those growing up in dysfunctional families.

Friendships

Friends are those we choose to develop close bonds with. They often become confidantes, advisors, and significant influences in our support system, especially during times of crisis, which arise for us all. Friends can provide a companionship and emotional stability that helps to reduce and manage depression, anxiety, and the many other mental conditions that can arise as we manage the complexities of modern life.

Romantic Relationships

Intimacy is essential for all humans. Loving passionately and being loved back in equal measure is like discovering and sharing an oasis of connection and happiness midst this complex world. Healthy romantic relationships can also help give our lives more purpose and meaning, when we share our life direction with someone and learn how to support each other's growth. Studies have proven that people in positive romantic relationships enjoy greater mental and physical health benefits than those who are not.

Professional Relationships

These play a powerful role in strengthening our sense of wellbeing during the working week. Relationships with colleagues, supervisors, mentors and clients, they can give us a sense of "family" but in our careers. Positive professional relationships also empower our sense of purpose, fulfillment, and expansion as we grow our careers. Supporting each other, professionally, enables all of us to develop skills, knowledge, and expertise more rapidly. Good professional relationships can also provide a different kind of emotional support, through the guidance and mentorship integral to professional growth and development. Studies have revealed that those in relationships that foster personal wellbeing enjoy higher job satisfaction ratings, superior mental health, and an enhanced sense of wellbeing than those without such support networks in place.

Community Relationships

These can include neighbors, community leaders, or those we meet through the activities of our children (other parents, teachers and coaches, etc.). Positive community relationships expand our range of relationship skills, as we relate to strangers who can become friends and allies. Studies have indicated that individuals who engage in supportive and positive interactions beyond family and work enjoy better mental and physical wellbeing than those without those extended connections.

Well established, supportive community relationships prove vital when dealing with serious disease. Having an available network can make a big difference for recovery. A disruptive health challenge is always physically, mentally, and emotionally draining so having reliable friends by your side is beyond essential. Without my friends and family, it would have been impossible for me to survive my catastrophic health challenges and what we encountered with my two children.

Self-Test: How Strong Are Your Relationship Skills?

Do you want to find out how well you can improve your relationships and create a reliable support network? Here's a fun self-test to help you discover your relationship strengths! For each question, choose the answer that best represents your current situation and behaviors. Write down the five numbers and then record your answer next to each one, a – c.

1. **Go-to Support** a) I have a solid support system in place, with someone to rely on during challenging times. b) I have a few friends I can count on, but I'm not always comfortable asking for help. c) I often feel alone and unsure where to turn when I need support.
2. **Practical Assistance** a) I have friends and family members who willingly offer practical assistance when I'm in need. b) I tend to handle most things on my own, but I know a few people who might help if I asked. c) I rarely ask for help with daily tasks, even when it's challenging for me.
3. **Emotional Support** a) I have a strong emotional support network, including friends, family, and professionals. b) I have

some friends I can talk to, but I'm hesitant about opening up completely. c) I often feel isolated and struggle to express my emotions to others.
4. **Investment in Relationships** a) I actively nurture my relationships and have invested time in building a diverse support network. b) I maintain my existing relationships but I haven't actively expanded my support network. c) I've neglected my relationships and I rarely seek out new connections.
5. **Proactive Approach** a) I believe in preparing for the future and establishing a support network before I need it. b) I'm somewhat aware of the importance of a support network but haven't taken significant steps to build one. c) I usually react to crises as they happen and haven't thought much about creating a support network in advance.

Scoring:
- For every "a" answer, give yourself 2 points.
- For every "b" answer, give yourself 1 point.
- For every "c" answer, give yourself 0 points.

Interpretation:
- 8-10 points: You're a Relationship Rockstar! You have a strong support network and understand the importance of nurturing relationships.
- 5-7 points: You're on the Right Track! You have some aspects of a support network but could work on strengthening it.
- 0-4 points: Time to Invest! Building a reliable support network could significantly improve your relationships and overall well-being.

Remember, relationships are an ongoing journey and there's always room for improvement. Use your results as a starting point to enhance your support network and create stronger connections with others.

According to extensive research, having an efficient support network plays an essential role in optimizing treatment results and decreasing complications. Establishing that network should be done before a crisis develops. Relationships take time to develop but this is a great investment. Your network should consist of friends and family as well as medical professionals, to ease a difficult journey and make things simpler for all concerned.

Turning An Enemy into a Friend

Your worst relationship is often with yourself.

Most of us have an inner critic who nags at us with whispered discouragement, like a dog nipping at our heels. But we can flip the script on what that character has to say. It's not easy to silence those negative voices that are trying to derail you by criticizing, shaming, insulting, and judging you. Instead, learn to replace the negative judgment with positive appreciation.

No matter what health tools you might have at your disposal, without knowing how to overcome the influence of negative self-talk, it will prove challenging to achieve your health goals. Whether your goal is weight loss, living disease free, launching your dream project, or something else entirely, it's essential to know that you are in control, not that sabotaging inner voice.

We began exploring this in our description of Superpower #2, the relationship with yourself. I'm expanding the commentary here because it's so vitally important. So, how *do* you take charge of your self-talk? It starts with knowing that it's always happening and that you *can* control it. Negative self-talk is a habit, one that all of us have. But not all of us passively give in to it. We can take a stand, sometimes even being rude to that voice. "Shut up!" is an appropriate response to demeaning comments, like: "You can't do it. You've tried to lose weight for years. You've always failed, and you always will. Why don't you just give up right now. How about some ice cream? You deserve a treat."

If your "Shut up!" works, be ready with a positive comment and put it in the first tense so there's no "other" yapping at you. How about something like:

"I'm strong. No matter how hard this might get, I'm going to do it. I know I can. And being successful with this will change my whole life!"

Creating Your Healthy Relationship with Food

Yes, it *is* a relationship, an intimate one, one you invest in every day.

If your relationship with food already seems healthy, great. If not, we can change that right now. Good nutrition is superpower #5 but this is different; it's not about the food itself but your relationship with it.

First, let's consider what an ideal relationship with food is *not*. It's not being on a restrictive diet or depriving yourself of all of the things you love to eat. It's not about duty and sacrifice. It's not about shrinking from enjoyment. It *is* about understanding that your body needs certain nutrients to remain healthy and content, making a commitment to provide them, paying attention to the signals your body sends you, then responding with intelligence and enjoying the food your body is asking for, without feeling any guilt or shame.

Why does having a positive relationship with food matter so much?

Because it can turn theory into practice. You may know in theory that when your body receives the right vitamins and minerals from nutritious sources that all its functions will improve. You may know in theory that you will have more energy, that your immune system will become stronger, that chronic illnesses such as diabetes or cardiovascular disease could be significantly reduced and that maintaining a balanced diet will improve your overall wellbeing. You may even believe that healthy food choices will help your weight normalize.

You may know all that and more. But, are you acting on what you know? You will, if you've developed a healthy relationship with food. Just as with any other relationship that we make a commitment to, it's natural to feel motivated to contribute to the success of the relationship.

The starting point for building a better relationship with food is to understand that it's not first about the food itself. There's no single right approach, no perfect diet, no formula that works for everyone. What works for you may not work for your neighbor. And what works for you today, might not be as helpful in three months. The priority is actually committing to that relationship.

If you're married, remember how the proposal felt? Well, propose to your food relationship to establish an equally committed relationship!

You're not cheating on your spouse… don't cheat on your food.

Here are a few suggestions to get you started:

Pay attention to what your body tells you. When you are hungry, eat. Once you feel 80% full, stop. While this seems obvious, many of us have become so accustomed to disregarding our bodies' signals that we may ignore hunger, then fail to stop when we're full. With practice, however, you'll quickly learn how to tune in and fulfill your body's needs.

Focused eating will lead you toward enjoying it more while decreasing the chances of overeating. By being present and enjoying every moment, food mindfulness will help you enjoy more and avoid overindulgence.

Give yourself permission to enjoy food without guilt. Don't shame yourself if you enjoy a slice of cake or a small bag of chips now and then.

Just savor the experience before reconnecting with your establishing eating patterns.

What you eat 80% of the time is more important than what you eat 20% of the time.

Get creative in the kitchen! Cooking can become an engaging and enriching experience that helps build your appreciation of food. Explore new recipes and experiment with various flavors, spices, and ingredients and relish every step along the way.

Surround yourself with positive influences. Hanging out with people who are constantly talking about diets and weight loss may actually make it harder for you to develop an uplifting relationship with food. Prioritize friends and activities that embrace a wide perspective on what's required to be healthy, rather than focusing just on dieting.

Growing your healthy relationship with food takes practice and patience but with time and determination you can learn to enjoy food without a sense of obligation, guilt, or shame. When you do this, it will inspire family and friends to join the party. Here's one good news story about exactly that.

Jenny

Jenny decided to start a clean eating plan with me because she wanted to lose weight and become healthier. With my guidance, she began eating all kinds of vegetables, whole grains, and lean proteins. Her husband was less than thrilled.

Tom would gaze longingly into the refrigerator at a pizza box, or order takeout, while Jenny prepared, served up, and enjoyed healthy dishes like grilled chicken with steamed vegetables and curried rice in a bowl. Tom watched, amazed. He couldn't believe anyone would choose to eat what he thought was bland, tasteless food.

Jenny, however, was determined to adhere to her plan and refused to get discouraged by Tom's objections. She continued to prepare healthy meals every night, while Tom continued to complain and grumble.

One evening, something strange happened. Jenny prepared a stir-fry of vegetables with black rice and beef. Tom took a bite, reluctantly, expecting the worst (All "diet food" tasted terrible, he believed.).

To his surprise, it was delicious! He was shocked. The vegetables and beef were cooked perfectly and well-seasoned. The black rice was fluffy, flavorful and satisfying. Much to his surprise, he really enjoyed a healthy dinner!

From that moment on, Tom began to look at food very differently. He had just experienced for himself that healthy food did not have to taste like dry cardboard. It could be as tasty as his favorite takeout foods. He became excited to try the new recipes Jenny was learning and before long it was Jenny who was complaining – that Tom was eating all of the leftovers she had intended for her lunch.

And, of course, you know what happened, right ladies? Jenny lost weight. So did Tom, with little to no effort. The pounds were melting off fast. Jenny was thrilled, because now she had her husband's enthusiastic support to shop and cook healthy food. They even rid their home of junk food.

Tom's cholesterol went down and he began sleeping better. BTW, Tom wasn't my client, Jenny was. She got a two-for! When I speak to Jenny now, she often says something like, "whenever Tom sees me eating something he's not sure is healthy and thinks I'm cheating, he says WWSMD." This stands for What Would Sonia Marie Do???" He actually got this printed onto a sweatshirt for her as a Christmas present. She told me, "Our whole family uses this expression now and they're all changing their diets!"

There were other benefits. Their relationship deepened. Jenny and Tom learned to respect each other more, to work together to achieve all their shared goals, and even to enjoy cooking together.

Building Our Healthy Relationship with Food

Jenny and Tom's story illuminates the infectious nature of building a healthy relationship with food. Here are a few helpful strategies for optimizing that relationship:

1. Determine what your health goals are and why you want to achieve them.
2. Write them down.
3. Make a commitment. Ask, "What could stop me from reaching my goals?"
4. Connect with a "health buddy." Ask them to support you.
5. Start, then sustain momentum. Persisting can be difficult which is why it's so important to have your healthy support network in place before you start the new program.

It's a Bird, It's a Plane, It's…

Remember the old Superman tv show that began that way? I was a Wonder Woman fan! Either way, I'm sure we'd all like to be able to fly. I'm not talking about physical flying now, which we need an airplane to do. I'm referring to the feeling of soaring in our lives, feeling elevated above our problems and enjoying the view. This is something we do together and sharing a healthy relationship with our food gives us an ideal context for that.

You may be dubious, given how addicted we are in our culture to shared enjoyments that are harmful to our health – like drinking and partying to excess – but all I can say is you have to experience it to know it. Sharing a love for healthy food with those you love can become a great enjoyment in your life.

PART THREE

BECOMING WELL

CHAPTER 15

SAVORY RECIPES

"It's more important to understand the imbalances in your body's basic systems and restore balance, rather than name the disease and match the pill to the ill."

—Dr. Mark Hyman

When we've activated superpower number one—Life awareness—we become more attuned to the signals our body gives us about what kinds of foods we need. Physical and mental symptoms aren't just problems to fix but are potentially helpful indicators of deficiencies, stagnation, and depletion. They can guide us to heal our bodies.

When it comes to holistic nutrition, the real value resides in savory foods. Sweet flavors get our attention – "treats" are almost always sweet - but savory foods offer significantly greater health benefits. When we learn how to prepare them properly, they can easily become more desirable than sweet foods, even for treats.

"Regardless of their palates, there's still a number of things American snackers universally agree on. For 35 percent of the poll, the prime time for a snack is in the early afternoon."[25]

Why is that? Here's an answer from a recent article in Vogue magazine: "We've all been there before: It's 4:00 p.m., you've eaten

---

[25] https://studyfinds.org/sweet-savory-snack-personality/

lunch, but somehow you're hungry again and craving a sweet snack. A coffee just won't do it and the Milk Bar cake from a coworker's birthday celebration is calling your name. Oh, and so are the M&M's in the vending machine. Top it off with a handful of Twizzlers Bites from a nearby desk and suddenly you're buzzing and primed for a crash. But what if you could prevent these feelings—and the way they tend to derail your overall fitness goals—and stay completely satisfied from lunch until dinner?"[26]

The author goes on to recommend a substantial savory dish lunch. She writes, ""A lunch that combines fiber and protein will keep you full and happy all afternoon."

Savory Foods: Nutrient Powerhouses

When we hear the word "savory," we may automatically think of the rich and bold flavors associated with foods like as garlic, onions, and herbs. But "savory" is about much more than flavor and taste, savory foods are packed full of nutrients: proteins, healthy fats, and complex carbohydrates.

Savory foods *regulate* blood sugar levels, while sugary treats often cause spikes and crashes in blood sugar. This means that savory foods give us sustainable energy. How important is that!? They do this thanks to the fiber and protein content that slows the rate of absorption into our bloodstream.

Savory foods also contain powerful antioxidants that protect the body against oxidative stress and inflammation, something of great significance given that chronic inflammation is linked to numerous health conditions like heart disease, cancer, and diabetes.

---

[26] https://www.vogue.com/article/stop-sugar-cravings-resolutions

Savory Supports Gut Health

Savory foods provide an additional major advantage for our overall health by strengthening the gut microbiome, that collective of trillions of bacteria living inside us that contribute to our overall wellbeing in foundational ways. A strong gut microbiome is associated with enhanced immunity, improved digestion, and even greater mental wellbeing.

Savory foods support a healthy gut microbiome in many ways. First, many savory foods are high in fiber which feeds beneficial bacteria living in the gut, and some also contain probiotics, live bacteria which help improve gut health and should become part of our daily diet.

Fermented foods like kimchi and sauerkraut, bone broth, and dark leafy greens are among the best savory foods for gut health, providing essential nutrients while supporting a thriving gut microbiome.

Foods With Flavor For Weight Loss

If you're trying to lose weight, savory foods must become the invaluable centerpiece of your diet. They contain high amounts of protein which will help you feel full and satisfied more quickly. Many savory dishes also register with a low caloric intake, which makes them ideal substitutes for more calorically dense snacks and desserts like chips and candy.

Many studies have demonstrated that people who consume savory foods like avocado and nuts tend to snack less on unhealthy food later in the day due to how these savory foods regulate their blood sugar levels ... which satisfies those cravings.

Savory Foods Heal the Body

Delicious savory foods can quickly become invaluable for your healing. Garlic and onion both contain compounds with proven antibacterial, antiviral, and anti-inflammatory properties. Turmeric - another tasty spice - has been touted for its ability to decrease inflammation while supporting joint health.

Leafy greens and cruciferous vegetables contain many essential vitamins and minerals for overall health, helping to reduce the risk of chronic disease while supporting natural healing processes in your body.

We know that food is medicine. The foods we eat promote either health or disease. We also know that it's important to select the *right* healthy foods for our unique bodies, that there is no ideal diet or health regime that delivers optimal health to everyone.

> *We must become detectives, sleuthing our way to the perfect food choices for us.*

If that sounds daunting, let's get motivated by reviewing a few compelling benefits:

1. Anti-inflammatory substances are abundant in these products. Especially garlic, turmeric, and ginger reduce inflammation and relieve pain in the body. Chronic inflammation is linked to many health problems, such as autoimmune diseases and heart disease. Adding more anti-inflammatory foods to your diet also improves overall health.
2. Supports immune function. Many foods rich in vitamins, minerals, and fiber, like leafy greens and mushrooms, support the health of the immune system, which boosts your body's defenses against disease and illness, making you more resistant to infection and accelerating your healing processes.
3. Regulates blood sugar levels. The complex carbohydrates found in savory foods can help to regulate blood sugar levels, preventing spikes and energy crashes. Choosing unprocessed, whole foods like sweet potato and brown rice and quinoa helps prevent developing insulin resistance.

4. Healthy fats. Nuts, avocados, and seeds are rich in healthy fats. These fats help to reduce inflammation, promote brain function, and help to maintain healthy skin, hair, and nails.
5. Protein. The body needs protein to build and repair tissues. Protein-rich foods like meat, fish, and legumes support muscle repair and growth. Protein is also essential for the immune system and helps you feel full between meals.

> *Choosing more healthy savory foods is one of the best primary strategies for improving your health. Turn them into treats and reap the benefits!*

As a functional medicine chef, my goal in working with clients is to teach them how to craft delicious, nutrient-dense meals that support healing and sustain optimal health. Activate superpower number five, good nutrition, to make your treats of choice savory rather than sweet and discover for yourself just how delicious savory can be. Here are some quick and easy and delicious recipes to help you heal from within.

Turmeric Roasted Vegetables

To make turmeric-roasted vegetables, simply toss your favorite veggies with coconut or avocado oil and turmeric powder and add a little salt before roasting in the oven until tender. Carrots, sweet potatoes, broccoli, cauliflower, and Brussel sprouts are ideal ingredients.

Salmon and Sweet Potato Bowl

To create the ultimate salmon and sweet potato bowl, bake a sweet potato, then layer on cooked salmon, steamed vegetables, and a drizzle of tahini sauce for the perfect salmon and sweet potato combo.

Quinoa and Lentil Salad

Quinoa and lentils are packed with protein and fiber. They are also low on the Glycemic Food Index Scale and will help you feel full and satisfied without triggering blood sugar spikes and crashes. To create a quinoa and lentil salad, simply cook according to package directions,0 then combine with chopped vegetables, herbs, and an easy dressing consisting of olive oil, lemon juice, and Dijon mustard for a delicious dish.

Garlic and Ginger Chicken Stir-Fry

To create this dish, sauté chopped garlic and ginger with chopped chicken pieces in coconut oil until tender before stirring in your choice of veggies. Stir-fry until done. Enjoy over brown or cauliflower rice as an ideal healthy and satisfying entree.

Roasted Beet and Goat Cheese Salad

Beets are packed with antioxidants that support liver health. To create this salad, simply roast beets in the oven until tender before cutting them into slices and combining with crumbled goat cheese, over mixed greens, with an easy dressing made from olive oil, balsamic or apple cider vinegar, and Dijon mustard.

Cauliflower Pizza

Cauliflower makes for an excellent low-carb alternative to the wheat in traditional pizza crusts and is full of vitamins and minerals. To create one, pulse cauliflower florets in a food processor until they resemble rice before mixing with eggs and your desired seasonings, then bake in the oven until crispy. Add your favorite cheese toppings; the healthiest are whole fat mozzarella in brine, goat cheese, and feta.

Chickpea and Spinach Curry

Chickpeas are an excellent plant-based source of protein that can help regulate blood sugar levels, while spinach provides essential vitamins and minerals for immune support.

To create this dish, sauté onions, garlic, and ginger in coconut oil before adding canned organic chickpeas, fresh tomatoes, and spinach. Simmer until the flavors have combined into an appetizing, energizing, filling meal. Serve over brown rice or quinoa.

My Favorite Mac-n-Cheese

Use a gluten free or bean pasta and make according to the package directions. For the cheesy sauce, boil three white potatoes with three sweet potatoes medium size and, once they are cooked through, blend with one tsp of powdered mustard, one tbsp of nutritional yeast, one tsp of turmeric, garlic and onion powder, plus just a dash of apple cider vinegar. Add in a cup of raw cashews (soaked for 15 minutes in hot water beforehand).

These are just a few examples of tasty and nutrient-dense savory entrees that are delicious and promote optimal health. Remember, while sweet foods tend to get more of the spotlight, savory ones are essential in contributing to overall health and well-being. Exercise your nutrition superpower and before long your taste buds will be begging you for savory snacks. They will quickly eclipse your past favorite sweet treats for pure flavor appeal and the health benefits will keep you motivated to continue "crowding out" the sweet with the savory.

Even your kids will enjoy this but don't tell them about the ingredients until they taste how irresistible it tastes!

CHAPTER 16

SWEET CAN BE GOOD

"All you need is love. But a little chocolate now and then doesn't hurt."

—Charles M. Schulz

Our bodies are constantly sending us signals about what they require, often as hunger, thirst, or fatigue. These cravings give us helpful clues about what our bodies need. As a holistic coach for the past 31 years, I've learned that most of my clients struggle with sugar cravings. But interpreting cravings properly can be a great way to understand what our bodies need.

Sometimes we do crave something sweet. Sweet cravings can indicate a number of things. Perhaps your body needs certain nutrients it is deficient in, or it could mean you need energy.

Lack of energy is one common cause for sweet cravings because sugar can provide a quick energy source for our bodies when we are rundown. When we are tired our appetite increases by about 25%. But eating sugar or carb-bage is only a temporary solution and it quickly leaves us feeling even more tired. The solution? Try fueling your body with whole foods that provide sustained energy. Nuts, seeds, and whole grains contain complex carbohydrates that will help you feel energized and full.

A lack of essential nutrients can also cause sweet cravings. If you crave chocolate, for example, this could be a sign that your body needs magnesium. Magnesium is a mineral that is vital for a number of bodily functions including muscle and nerve, heart, and bone health. Foods rich in magnesium include nuts, leafy greens, and whole grains. When you are including enough of foods that are rich in nutrients that support your body, you can also satisfy your sweet tooth.

Stress is another common cause of sweet cravings. Sugar can be a comforting and soothing substance for our bodies when we are stressed or anxious. But this can develop into a vicious circle of stress / sugar addiction. Instead of just reaching for something sweet, try incorporating stress-reduction practices into your everyday routine to break this cycle. Yoga, meditation, and deep breathing are all helpful. You can also support your body better by eating more whole foods rich in omega-3 fatty acid and B vitamins, in other words, savory foods.

Sweet – The Good, The Bad, The Ugly

Not all sweet foods are the same. Some are actually rich in nutrients and provide energy. Others, however, contain empty calories and cause weight gain, chronic disease, inflammation, and other health problems. Here are general categories of healthy sweet food choices:

- Fresh fruit is an excellent source of fiber, vitamins, and antioxidants. Add fresh fruit to meals and snacks to give them a sweet boost.
- Nuts & seeds: Nuts & seeds are high in fiber, healthy fats and protein. They can keep you satisfied and full. Many nuts taste slightly sweet, which can satisfy your sugar cravings.
- Dark chocolate: Dark chocolate contains antioxidants. Choose chocolate with at least 72% cocoa to reap the maximum health benefits.

- Sweet vegetables. Vegetables such as sweet potatoes, beets, carrots and other root crops can have a natural sweetness and provide vitamins and minerals. Roasting vegetables with olive oil and salt makes a tasty and satisfying side dish.

We can satisfy our sweet cravings while also nourishing the body by tuning in to these cravings and choosing foods that promote our health and energy.

The good – whole foods with a sweet taste.
The bad – sweet treats full of empty calories.
The ugly – heavily processed candy, full of chemicals.

Sweet foods may seem indulgent and unhealthy, but I believe they have their place in a nutritious diet. In fact, when consumed mindfully and in moderation they provide important health benefits. Here are eight examples of sweet foods that support health while satisfying those cravings.

Dark chocolate is a tasty treat with many health advantages. Packed with antioxidants and flavonoids that can reduce inflammation and lower blood pressure, dark chocolate also boosts serotonin levels to improve mood and decrease stress levels. Choose dark chocolate that contains at least 72% cacao for optimal health benefits.

Berries are an extremely tasty and nutritional fruit, low glycemic, with ample antioxidant benefits. Anthocyanins present in berries have been proven to reduce inflammation while simultaneously improving brain function. Plus, berries provide added fiber that aids digestion while providing lasting satisfaction.

Honey has been used as a natural sweetener and medicine for many centuries. Loaded with antioxidants and antimicrobial compounds that boost immune function and fight off infections, honey can also improve sleep quality in children who suffer from upper respiratory infections as well as reduce coughing symptoms and lessen seasonal allergies. Buy local honey from your farmers' market. This can make a significant impact on your seasonal allergies because the bees in your area will give you the immunities your body needs to address the allergies in your environment.

Dates are an abundant source of fiber, vitamins, and minerals that help promote overall health and bone development. They contain potassium, magnesium, and iron which have been shown to lower blood pressure. Furthermore, dates provide antioxidant protection which may reduce inflammation as well as the risk for chronic diseases. Just two dates a day can help in weight loss for women over 45.

Sweet potatoes are an abundant and nutritious root vegetable full of essential vitamins and minerals. Sweet potatoes contain beta-carotene which the body converts into vitamin A to improve vision while strengthening immunity and providing benefits like improved eyesight and immune support. Sweet potatoes also contain fiber which aids digestion and promotes feelings of fullness and that supports weight control. Sweet potatoes are my number one weight loss superfood.

Cinnamon is an aromatic spice with many health advantages. Packed with antioxidants and anti-inflammatory compounds, cinnamon is known to reduce inflammation and the risk of chronic diseases while improving blood sugar control and insulin sensitivity. Cinnamon also boosts metabolism, which makes it an excellent choice for those living with diabetes or insulin resistance.

Apples are an abundant source of fiber and antioxidants, helping reduce inflammation while decreasing risk for chronic diseases. Apples provide vitamin C which supports immunity and maintains skin health. In my holistic world, we call apples natures caffeine because apples give you a lift in energy.

Maple syrup is an amazing natural sweetener full of antioxidants and minerals that support immune health. It's high in zinc, which supports immune health and manganese, which helps manage blood sugar levels. Maple syrup also contains polyphenols which may reduce inflammation and decrease the risk of chronic diseases.

Bonus Sweetener: Black Strap Molasses is naturally rich in antioxidants, iron, calcium, magnesium, potassium, phosphorus, and vitamin B6. It may relieve constipation, help treat anemia, and support bone and hair health.

Easy Peasy

I don't believe that eating delicious, nutritious desserts needs to be time-consuming or complicated. Here are eight quick and easy recipes for sweets that will satisfy your palate and improve your health.

1. Chocolate Banana Smoothie Bowl - Blend frozen bananas with almond milk, cacao, and your favorite protein powder. Pour into a large bowl, top with banana slices, cacao nibs, and almond butter.
2. Vanilla Chia pudding: Combine chia seeds with almond milk, vanilla, maple syrup, and vanilla extract in a mason-jar. Shake well, and place in the refrigerator for an hour or more. Serve with fresh berries, and sliced almonds.
3. Cinnamon-Roasted Sweet Potatoes: Cut the sweet potatoes into bite sized pieces, then toss them with coconut oil and cinnamon. Add a pinch of salt. Roast sweet potatoes in the oven, until they are tender and caramelized. Serve as a dessert or a side. Top with coconut whipped cream.
4. Almond Butter Stuffed dates: Cut the dates in half and remove the pit. Spread almond butter in each half and sprinkle with sea salt. You can even dip them in melted chocolate. You're welcome!!!!
5. Layer Greek yogurt with mixed berries and gluten-free granola in a tall glass. Add a drizzle of cinnamon and honey on top.

6. Caramelized Pear Salad with Walnuts: Slice the pears, then toss them in Ghee or coconut oil, balsamic, and maple syrup. Roast until caramelized and tender. Serve over arugula, with goat cheese crumbles and toasted nuts.
7. Coconut Flour Pancakes - Mix coconut flour, almond milk and vanilla extract with a little honey. Cook on a nonstick pan until each side is golden brown. Serve with fresh berries and maple syrup drizzled on top.
8. Date ginger cookies - my favorite. I will save this recipe for our last chapter!

These are just a few of the many recipes that can satisfy your sweet tooth and still help you maintain a balanced, healthy diet. Enjoy!

Sweet foods have an important place in a balanced and healthy diet when eaten mindfully and in moderation. When selecting sweets, look for less processed options with nutrients that support optimal health, remembering that having an assortment of food sources is the key to optimal wellness!

In the next chapter I will be sharing my favorite recipes for Life, ranging from hearty soups and stews to vibrant salads and stir-fries. Food plays such a critical role in overall wellness. What we eat has an enormous influence over physical, mental and emotional wellbeing. I am proud to introduce to you these recipes which provide delicious, healthy, sustainable options to nourish both body and mind.

No matter your experience level in the kitchen, these recipes offer something for every cook, from novices to master chefs alike. These user-friendly recipes will inspire healthy living habits for lifelong success and happiness.

I'm so glad you're accompanying me on my culinary journey and discovering just how delicious and rewarding a holistic, sustainable, functional medicine lifestyle can be!

CHAPTER 17

RECIPES FOR LIFE

"Reading a book, for me at least, is like traveling in someone else's world. If it's a good book, then you feel comfortable and yet anxious to see what's going to happen to you there, what'll be around the next corner."

—Jonathan Carroll

Congratulations! Here we are, in the last chapter. What's next for you? It's time to put what you've read and learned into practice. I've given you recipes for life, enough for a virtual lifetime of exploration, not just in the kitchen but in the *whole* of your life. We've been exploring your seven healing superpowers, hopefully in a way that will help you continue to activate these powers throughout every aspect of your life.

Here's the one simple but profound idea which perfectly describes the mindset of "being well:"

Every choice contributes to improving our health ... or not.

This explains why, of all the superpowers, we place choice in the middle. We use that superpower to determine which of the others we activate.

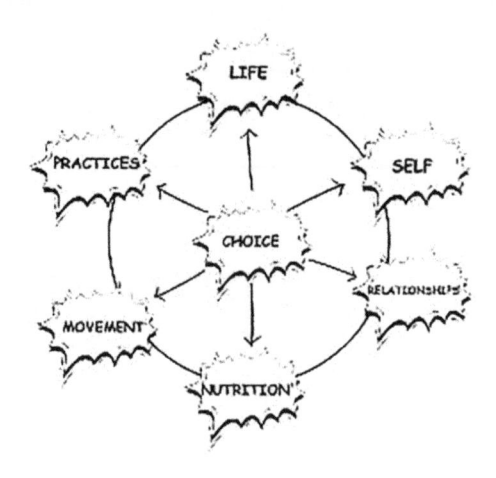

In this last chapter, I match one recipe with each of the superpowers, we give it a memorable name, identify the healing properties of one of the ingredients, and connect with the healing property of what you'll prepare. The result, I hope, is that you will begin to consider what to eat in a very different way. As I said earlier, we are what we eat… and much more. I'm choosing to emphasize this fifth superpower, nutrition, as one very practical way to integrate this new habit of choosing to be well.

Speaking of choices, what's in a name?

Marketers will tell you: everything! Menu experts point out the obvious, that the name of a dish should tell you something about it. But it should also fascinate. Devoting a few minutes of creative thought to naming what you're preparing shows how much you care about it, that you're not just casually making something, and then serving it up, end of story.[4]

An inventive name creates mystique, it adds to the appeal, you might even say that it begins the digestive process early, by stimulating anticipation. Remember Pavlov's famous experiment where he demonstrated how dogs, who salivated when they were fed, could be trained to salivate when they heard a bell announcing that food was coming?

How you name your personal menu items can have that same effect. Imagine calling your family for dinner. As they arrive and ask, "What's for dinner?" you say, "Salad, fish, and potatoes." They probably won't be jumping up and down with enthusiasm when they hear that. But what if you answered, "Blissful Peach & Tomato Salad with Wild Cod and Mini Potatoes in a Miracle Medley." Say, what? Now, that's going to catch their attention!

So, here are seven dishes with cool names. I've assembled the full recipes and details on nutritional benefits into a companion e-book, free on my website, https://www.soniamarienutrition.com

Superpower One - Life

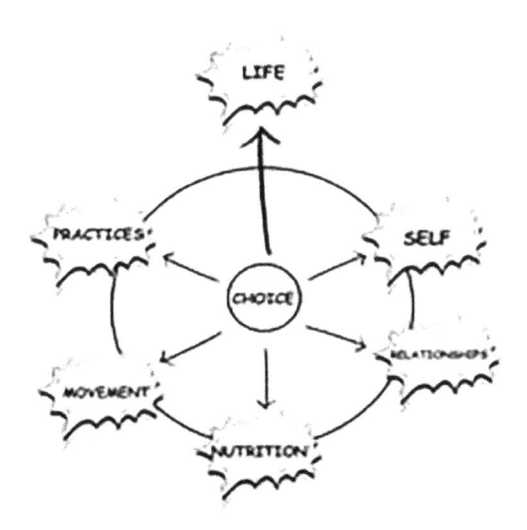

Eternal Essence Elixir

This delicious drink makes for a wonderful breakfast or afternoon snack. As you sip, think about what a miracle your life is and enjoy the feeling of gratitude as you savor this blockbuster supercharger!

Ingredients: Water, Cacao Powder, Maple Syrup, Sea Salt, Maca Powder, Lion's Mane Powder, Oat Milk, Cinnamon.

Key Ingredient: Cacao Powder

Cacao, the blissful superfood derived from the cocoa bean, offers a wealth of health benefits. Rich in antioxidants, it nurtures our cells, offering protection from oxidative stress and inflammation. Its natural compounds also promote cardiovascular health, support cognitive function, and elevate mood by boosting the production of feel-good neurotransmitters like serotonin and endorphins. But the value of cacao extends far beyond its alluring flavor, it's also a vibrant elixir for your heart's well-being.

Deep within its own healing heart, cacao harbors an abundance of flavonoids, those awe-inspiring antioxidants engaged in an intimate affair with your cardiovascular system. With each sumptuous encounter, these flavonoids nourish your blood vessels, sustaining flexibility and healthy blood flow. Your heart, beating to the rhythm of life itself, is nourished by cacao's affection, enveloped in a tapestry of vitality that echoes through every beat.

Scan this code (insert) to receive my free e-book for this recipe and the other six in this last chapter. Or visit my website: https://www.soniamarienutrition.com

Superpower Two - Self

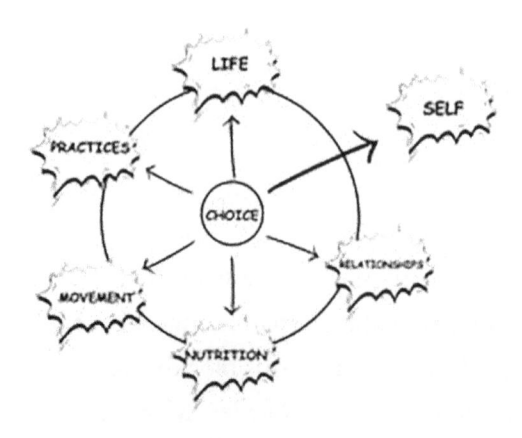

Soulful Serenity Soup

Let the comforting warmth of this Soulful Serenity Soup envelop your senses, inviting a profound sense of contentment in just being yourself. From the very first spoonful, you can anticipate a wave of soothing tranquility washing over you as the worries of your day simply melt away, replaced by a profound enjoyment of total self-care. This soup is much more than a meal, it's a mindfulness experience, savoring the delicious serenity of the present, one spoonful at a time.

Ingredients: Diced Tomatoes, Chickpeas, Dry Lentils, Onions, Celery, Green Bell Pepper, Parsley, White Onion, Ginger, Cumin, Saffron, Chili Powder, Sea Salt, Turmeric, Cinnamon, Black Pepper, Brown Rice, Vegetable Stock, Coconut Oil.

Key Ingredient: Saffron

Yes, it has a beautiful hue. But did you know that saffron contains antioxidants that protect the body from oxidative stress and inflammation, supporting mental clarity and emotional well-being? This precious spice, extracted from the heart of these blooms, holds within it the power to illuminate your emotions. Saffron is like a gentle alchemist. It interacts with your brain, stimulating the release of neurotransmitters that can paint your inner canvas with shades of serenity and contentment.

Superpower Three - Relationships

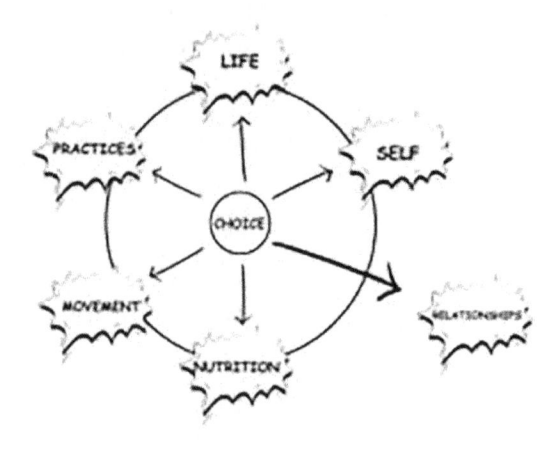

Blissful Peach & Tomato Salad

Indulge in the exquisite flavors of this Blissful Peach & tomato salad as it transports you into pure culinary delight. Each bite becomes a harmonious dance between the juicy sweetness of ripe peaches and the vibrant freshness of plump tomatoes. Know that as you savor this salad you are nurturing a beautiful relationship between your taste buds and the bountiful gifts of nature. Allow the crispness of the greens to caress your senses and remind you of the nurturing embrace of a loving relationship, where every moment carries the potential for experiencing pure bliss.

Ingredients: Peaches, Cherry Tomatoes, Red Onions, Feta Cheese, Extra Virgin Olive Oil, Raw Honey, Sea Salt, Basil Leaves

Key ingredient: Basil Leaves

With their refreshing aroma and vibrant green color, basil leaves offer a wealth of essential nutrients like vitamins A, K, and C, as well as magnesium and calcium. These nutrients support bone health, boost the immune system, and provide. valuable antioxidants for cellular protection. Compounds like the eugenol and polyphenols in basil contribute to improved digestion by enhancing enzymatic activity and promoting the balance of gut bacteria to aid in auto-immune health. These elements facilitate smoother nutrient absorption, reducing the likelihood of digestive discomfort. Incorporating basil into your meals is a step toward fostering a balanced and thriving gut environment, where the intricate dance of digestion lays the groundwork for optimal health.

Superpower Four – Choice

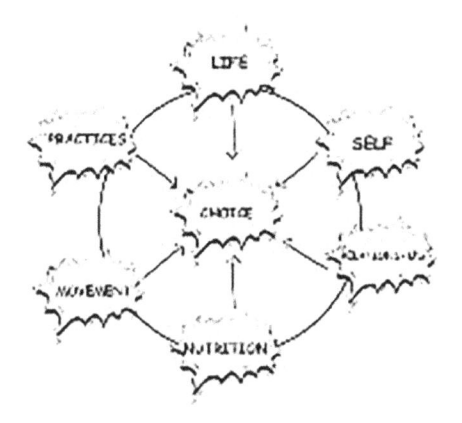

Wild Cod and Mini Potatoes Miracle Medley

Embark on a sensory journey of nourishment and delight with our wild cod and mini potatoes Miracle Melody. Each tender morsel of cod and every golden mini potato offers a testament to the exquisite choices that nature provides. As you savor this orchestra of flavors, remember that every bite is a choice for nurturing your well-being. Let this dish be a reminder that in every moment, we so have this choice, to actively nourish your body and soul.

Ingredients: Mini Potatoes, Extra Virgin Olive Oil, Lemon Juice, Sea Salt, Black Pepper, Cod Fillets, Zucchini, Capers, Fresh Dill

Key ingredient: Lemon Juice

A burst of citrus freshness, lemon juice offers a wealth of health benefits. High in vitamin C, it boosts our immune system, promotes collagen production, and aids in iron absorption. The alkalizing effect of lemon juice also supports the body's natural pH levels. Lemon, with its low glycemic index and citric acid content, can aid in stabilizing blood sugar levels after meals. This helps prevent rapid spikes and crashes, promoting sustained energy and reducing the risk of insulin resistance. Additionally, lemon's fiber content supports a feeling of fullness, potentially aiding in weight management efforts by curbing excessive eating.

Superpower Five – Nutrition

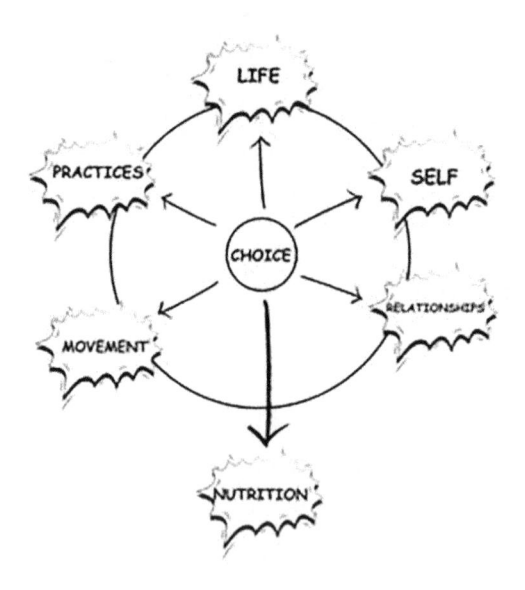

Irresistible Flourless Pancake Supreme

Indulge yourself! Our irresistible, flourless pancake Supreme is a healthy creation,where nutrition meets love in every delectable bite. These pancakes prove that nutritious eating can be an absolute delight, a comforting embrace for your taste buds *and* your well-being. Enjoy every guilt-free bite, relishing how taking care of yourself can taste this amazing! Nurturing body and soul this way is an easy choice to make!

Ingredients: All Natural Almond Butter, Unsweetened Almond Milk, Eggs, Baking Powder, Coconut Oil (for the pan), Protein Powder.

Key ingredient: Natural Almond Butter:

A wholesome and nutrient-dense spread, natural almond butter is a rich source of heart-healthy monounsaturated fats. These healthy fats support cardiovascular health and contribute to improved cholesterol levels.

Additionally, almond butter provides protein, fiber, vitamin E, and magnesium. Almond butter, like a warm embrace for your heart, holds a secret that can uplift your well-being. Packed with monounsaturated fats, it's a loyal companion to your cardiovascular health, gently working to balance cholesterol levels and support the delicate dance of blood circulation. As you savor its velvety goodness, know that you're nurturing a heartwarming relationship with your own body. It's a reminder that self-care can be as simple and delightful as spreading a dollop of almond butter on your morning toast, confirming the profound connection between the nourishment you receive and the wellness you experience.

Superpower Six - Movement

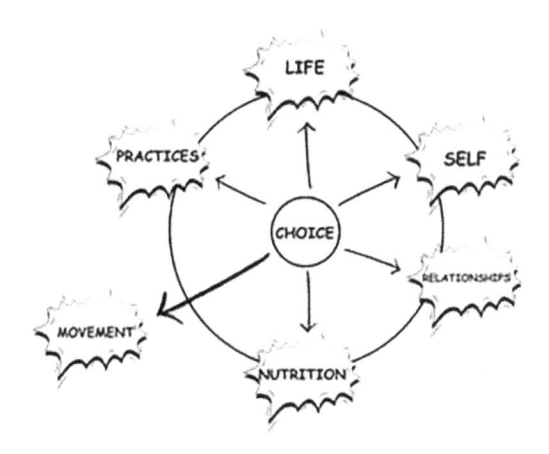

Delicata Squash & Cranberries Delight

As you savor the meaty squash and juicy burst of cranberries, you can literally feel the vitality they are infusing within your body. This dish is a reminder that the rhythm of life is like a dance, and just as the ingredients come together in harmony, so too can our bodies and souls when we embrace the joy of movement. Nurturing yourself with this delightful combination is not only a dining pleasure, but also an invitation to savor the beautiful synchrony of nourishment and movement in your life.

Ingredients: Delicata Squash, Frozen Cranberries, Extra Virgin Olive Oil, Maple Syrup, Cinnamon, Sea Salt, Goat Cheese, Pumpkin Seeds

Key ingredient -Pumpkin Seeds

Tiny but mighty, pumpkin seeds are a nutritional powerhouse, overflowing with protein, magnesium, and zinc. These seeds support immune function, promote heart health and provide nourishment for healthy skin and hair. Pumpkin seeds are a natural source of plant-based protein, rich in essential amino acids that form the building blocks of muscle tissue. These amino acids support the body's ability to repair and regenerate muscle fibers after physical activity. By incorporating pumpkin seeds into your diet, you're providing your muscles with the raw materials they need to recover and grow. These fatty acids help manage post-exercise inflammation, promoting quicker recovery and reducing the risk of overtraining-related issues.

Superpower Seven – Practices

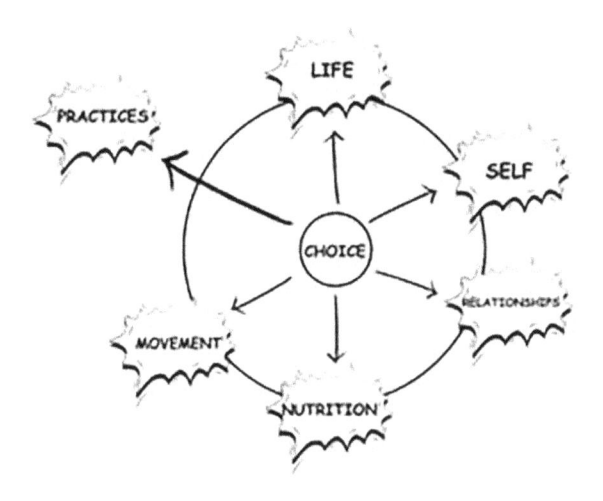

Dip of the Gods

Let the tantalizing aroma of This Dip of the Gods beckon you into a world of gastronomical delight. With every scoop, you will enjoy an explosion of flavors that nurture your taste buds *and* your soul. Why not make preparing and enjoying this dip a sacred ritual, one you can share with family and friends to remind everyone of the truly magical transformational process that eating and digesting is.

Ingredients: Extra Virgin Olive Oil, White Onion, Cumin Seed, Ginger, Garlic, Garam Masala, Fire Roasted Diced Tomatoes, Frozen Spinach, Plain Greek Yogurt, Water, Sea Salt, Paneer Cheese

Key Ingredient: Garam Masala

This aromatic spice blend combines various flavorful ingredients like cinnamon, cloves, and cardamom. Each component adds its unique health benefits, including antioxidant support and potential anti-inflammatory effects, contributing to holistic wellness. Garam Masala's blend of warming spices holds within it a treasure trove of compounds that aid digestion. Ingredients like cumin, coriander, and cardamom have been traditionally used to stimulate digestive enzymes, promoting efficient breakdown of nutrients. composition includes spices like black pepper, which contains piperine, known for its potential to boost metabolism. This spice blend, with its thermogenic properties, can contribute to increased calorie burning and energy expenditure.

By infusing your dishes with Garam Masala, you're engaging in a culinary strategy aligned with functional medicine principles, harnessing the power of metabolism to fuel your daily activities and amplify your overall energy levels.

In celebrating the interconnectedness of food and well-being, we embrace the inherent wisdom of whole foods and their profound impact on our journey to ultimate health and vitality. Nourishing our bodies with this delightful ensemble not only delights our senses but also nurtures our physical, emotional, and spiritual selves. With each lovingly prepared dish, we honor the essence of vibrant well-being and the beauty of embracing nature's bounty.

Appreciating Yourself

You did it! We did it! We made it to the end of the book. Let's celebrate… with one of these wonderful meals! Which one will you choose, and who will you invite to share it with you?

First, remember way back in Chapter Seven when I invited you to write a letter to yourself? Now is the time to either mail it, if you haven't already, or open it if you have.

As you read (wait until it arrives if you need to), connect with what you are feeling. How closely does it resemble what you imagined you'd be feeling back then and what you wrote in your letter?

Finish reading the letter and give yourself that big pat on the back, then choose the ideal way to celebrate, with one of these meals and some special friends.

I'd love to stay in touch and learn about your experience with these healing superpowers. I'm always available through my website and I'd love to send you the e-book I mentioned, where I provide more details on these seven dishes plus specific instructions on how to best prepare them.

Thank you once again for being my "client-by-book" and embracing this journey deep into the heart of being well!

Sonia Marie Romero

Finally, A Few Gifts:
https://www.soniamarienutrition.com/lead-collection

Youtube:
https://www.youtube.com/@soniamarienutrition9049/videos

Website:
https://www.soniamarienutrition.com/